"As a clinician who has worked with adrenally fatigued patients for more than fifteen years, this is the book I have been waiting for! This is a concise, practical guide for truly healing the adrenal glands. Not only does Kathryn Simpson provide an excellent in-depth section on the causes and symptoms of adrenal fatigue, she also clearly outlines the optimal diet, supplements, and herbs that can help reverse this condition. If you feel fatigued or burnt-out, follow the steps outlined in this guide and you will change your life! This is definitely a book I will recommend to my patients and to anyone suffering with this all-too-prevalent condition."

—Robin Marzi, RD, nutritional consultant

"After years of treating my patients with traditional therapies, I had the good fortune to meet Kathryn Simpson. After reviewing her extensive research and anecdotal experience, I decided to give hormonal treatment a try with my patients, and the results were amazing. Degenerative disease and even conditions like MS, fibromyalgia, and lupus responded to treating adrenal fatigue with bioidentical hormones and diet and lifestyle changes. Anyone with an inflammatory condition or disease should have their adrenal function tested. All it takes is a simple blood test."

—William B. Van Valin, II, MD, Chief of Staff,
Emeritus at Santa Ynez Valley Cottage Hospital

OVERCOMING

ADRENAL

FATIGUE

How to Restore Hormonal Balance *and* Feel Renewed, Energized, *and* Stress Free

KATHRYN R. SIMPSON, MS

New Harbinger Publications, Inc.

Normal cortisol production pattern Source: Kathryn Simpson, *The Women's Guide to Thyroid Health* (Oakland, CA: New Harbinger Publications, 2009).

The primary endocrine glands Source: Kathryn Simpson, *The Women's Guide to Thyroid Health* (Oakland, CA: New Harbinger Publications, 2009).

Thyroid stimulation pathway Source: Kathryn Simpson, *The Women's Guide to Thyroid Health* (Oakland, CA: New Harbinger Publications, 2009).

Distributed in Canada by Raincoast Books

Acquired by Melissa Kirk; Cover design by Amy Shoup; Edited by Jasmine Star

Library of Congress Cataloging-in-Publication Data on file with the publisher

14 13 12

10 9 8 7 6 5 4 3

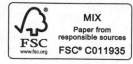

To my husband, Robert, and my sons, Tyler, Kyle, and Myles, who have steadfastly stuck by me through illness and the long hours of research my recovery has required, and who have had to hear more about adrenal function than anyone should have to!

Contents

Acknowledgments

To the many doctors who have generously collaborated with me over the years—to name a few, Thierry Hertoghe, William Van Valin, Victor Rosenfeld, Naomi Parry, Diana Schwarzbein, Guy Abraham, Scot Brewster, and Julie Taguchi.

To the many researchers who have advanced understanding of critical adrenal issues, and especially two of the best: Bruce McEwen, Ph.D., and Robert Sapolsky, Ph.D.

To Melissa Kirk and Jasmine Star at New Harbinger Publications for making this project possible, fun, and adrenal friendly.

To my colleagues and friends, especially Marian Lever, Ann Blumenthal, JoAnn Roland, Debbie Merino, Cathy Feldman, Liz Widdicombe, Kathryn Imani, Melissa Brewster, Margarita Lupin, Hiram French, and Lauren Otsuki.

And finally, to all the people with adrenal dysfunction who were willing to share their stories.

Foreword

Kathy Simpson has put her talents to work addressing a problem so many people suffer from and desperately seek help for: adrenal fatigue. The adrenals, two tiny endocrine glands located above the kidneys, exert a powerful influence on our lives. If they were to stop working completely, blood sugar levels would drop drastically and we would fall into a coma and die within twenty-four hours. But well before the situation reaches this point, the adrenals can become fatigued and lose function, bringing on a host of symptoms, from inflammation to irritability to an inability to tolerate even minor stress.

Kathy has a great advantage over many authors who write books on medical topics: She has inside knowledge, having once been afflicted with severe adrenal fatigue herself. Her firsthand knowledge is evident throughout the book.

Her book also has the merit of addressing factors beyond simply supplying the missing hormones. She gives clear information on critical approaches such as diet, nutritional supplements, adopting a healthier lifestyle, and cultivating positive thoughts. This book will be a valuable resource in helping you regain, and maintain, adrenal function and good health.

—Dr. Thierry Hertoghe
President of the International Hormone Society
Author of *The Hormone Handbook*, *The Patient Hormone Handbook*,
and *The Hormone Solution*

Introduction

Your adrenal glands can save your life—mine did. But it took me years to figure out the vital connection between my adrenal function and my health problems. I was diagnosed with multiple sclerosis (MS), a disease that's universally considered to be an inflammatory disease of the central nervous system. My diagnosis of MS was based on a roster of debilitating inflammatory symptoms: lesions in my brain and spinal column, elevated proteins in my spinal fluid, loss of eyesight, bladder problems, chronic fatigue, carpal tunnel syndrome, Bell's palsy, chronic back pain, irritable bowel syndrome, and more.

There were separate treatments for almost every symptom: medication for my pain and bladder problems, surgery for my hands, glasses for my vision, and on down the line. But never once did any of my doctors address the root cause of the inflammation that was attacking my system and how to resolve it.

My disease continued to progress, and I was running out of medical alternatives. Not being a doctor, I had no options other than to apply common sense to figuring out how to stop the disease's progression. I reasoned that if all my symptoms were linked to inflammation, then I had to find out how inflammation is created and managed within the body in order to stop it. I immersed myself in everything I could read, contacted everyone I knew in the scientific and medical communities, and eventually understood that my adrenal glands produced the critical hormones that control inflammation. I figured that something must be desperately wrong with mine and set out to resolve the problem.

Again, I turned to simple logic: Shouldn't it be easy to measure levels of these key hormones and supplement any that were deficient? When I took my research to a doctor friend, he felt it was compelling enough to give it a try. Sure enough, I was extremely deficient in cortisol, one of the primary hormones responsible for controlling inflammation in our bodies. Taking supplemental cortisol to get me back to healthy levels had an immediate effect on my symptoms. Within a short time after I started taking cortisol (as well as thyroid hormone therapy), every one of my inflammatory symptoms was gone! Nine years later, I'm still feeling great and am symptom free.

The first step in optimizing adrenal health is to get to the bottom of how your adrenal glands are currently functioning. The best way to start on this process is to evaluate your symptoms and, if they appear to be related to adrenal function, request that your doctor order tests to measure levels of key adrenal hormones. This book is designed to help you analyze these symptoms and decide on the best methods of testing for and treating adrenal dysfunction, based on the most up-to-date medical research.

The most common symptoms of low adrenal function are overwhelming fatigue and inability to handle stress. The complete list of possible symptoms of adrenal dysfunction is much more extensive and esoteric than most practitioners may realize. Here are just a few of the ways it may manifest:

- Excessive fatigue and exhaustion

- Low stamina

- Difficulty recovering from exercise

- Feeling run-down

- Feeling overwhelmed by or unable to cope with stress

- Craving salty and sweet foods

- Feeling most energetic in the evening

- Waking up tired, even after a full night's sleep

- Sleep disturbances

- Being slow to recover from stress, injury, or illness

- Difficulty concentrating

- Being highly susceptible to colds, flus, and infections

- Food or environmental allergies

- Premenstrual syndrome or unusually problematic menopause

- Consistent low blood pressure

- Extreme sensitivity to cold

There's no reason to suffer either the symptoms of adrenal hormone imbalance or the diseases they can lead to; you can't afford to passively sit by when it comes to your health.

It takes some work to get to the bottom of what's going on, but once you do, you'll have a clear picture of how your adrenals are functioning and whether they could be affecting your health and well-being. This is the information you'll need to chart your path to adrenal health. This book will give you the tools you need to detect and treat adrenal problems.

Here's to your good health!

CHAPTER 1

The Miraculous Adrenal Glands

Your adrenal glands are vital to your health and well-being. They help you survive stress by producing hormones that keep your body on an even keel despite the fact that you're constantly being buffeted by stressors you can't control. They help maintain homeostasis, bringing equilibrium to your energy level, your weight and body shape, your mind, your emotions, and just about every physiological system in your body.

When I use the word "stress," I'm not talking about just a bad day. I'm talking about the cumulative effects of a wide variety of situations: problems at work, at home, or within the family; worry, frustration, and inability to cope; and everything from long-term financial pressures or rush hour traffic to physical stressors like injury, infection, illness, inadequate diet, environmental toxins, or lack of sleep or exercise. Stress can be any external force that puts pressure on your mind or your body, and it can even include positive events, like marriage, a promotion, the birth of a baby, or moving to a new neighborhood or town.

The adrenals respond to any form of stress with a programmed biochemical response: the *stress response*, or, more popularly, the *fight-or-flight reaction*. When you experience stress, the adrenals release stress hormones—*cortisol* and *adrenaline*. This makes you extraordinarily alert.

Heart rate, breathing rate, blood pressure, and metabolism all speed up to increase the flow of oxygen and deliver it to muscles. Pupils dilate to sharpen vision. The liver releases stored blood sugar to increase energy. Sweat is produced to cool the body. The immune system goes on red alert, pumping out proinflammatory substances to attack invading bacteria and viruses and heal wounds and moving immune cells into their fighting positions.

Activities that aren't important to survival are immediately curtailed, such as blood flow to nonessential areas, including the hands, feet, scalp, and intestines. Blood vessels in the skin are also constricted, to lessen bleeding in case of injury, and blood clotting is increased to further control blood loss. Digestion is slowed so that the body can redirect its resources to deal with the stressor. And finally, natural painkillers are released to prevent the pain that could slow you down if you're injured.

MODERN STRESS

Historically, the stress response was geared to handling short-term events—crises that came and went quickly. Its purpose was to prepare us for a fight with a neighboring tribe or a quick dash to safety. We've all read stories about a parent being able to lift a car off a child. This short-lived super-human strength is fueled by adrenaline. It helped our ancestors survive encounters with ferocious beasts or hostile fellow humans. Those who survived such encounters often had time to recover from the exertion or any wounds sustained, allowing the adrenals to rest and recuperate.

Today our stressors are different—they're as often psychological as they are physical, and they don't seem to let up. We all know what modern stress feels like; we're inundated with it on any given day: *Rushing to get the kids ready for school, you cut your hand while slicing a bagel. You wrap it in gauze and head out the door. You drop the kids at school and head to work, catching up on calls while en route. Once there, you face nonstop meetings, calls, and presentations, and lunch is an energy bar and a diet cola. You navigate bumper-to-bumper traffic as you go to pick the kids up from after-school activities and stop for groceries on the way home. You walk in the door, make dinner, supervise homework, put the kids to bed, respond to e-mails, and then edit a spreadsheet for your client meeting first thing in the morning. You're lucky if you're in bed by midnight. Whew!*

Unfortunately, the body's response to this new kind of stress is the same as it was when our ancestors were fighting for their lives. Your body wants to survive the perceived threat, so it bypasses your brain to respond with the biological stress response.

Persistent stress causes your adrenal glands to constantly produce an excess of the stress hormones cortisol and adrenaline. Chronic exposure to these hormones suppresses healing and growth and can eventually cause problems with the many functions that are affected by the stress response, including digestion, energy, immunity, cognition, emotions, and metabolism.

COPING WITH MODERN STRESS

The modern stress situation isn't all gloom and doom, though: some mental stress can be a good thing. It can motivate us to productive action. It can excite us and enhance our sensory awareness and mental acuity. And if you understand how your body responds to stress, you can begin to control your physical reaction to it. One way to impact your body's response to stress to is make changes to your diet and lifestyle. The amount of sleep and exercise you get plays a part in your ability to handle stress, as does your use of substances like nicotine, drugs, and alcohol. In addition, your mental attitude can temper your physical reaction to stress.

Chapters 7 and 8 will discuss these factors in detail, but because your outlook can have such a profound impact on your stress response, it's worth spending a bit of time on this topic at the outset. In short, your physical reaction to stress is partially based on your interpretation of whether something is dangerous or not. This plays a large role in determining whether you will respond calmly or in full-on fight-or-flight mode—complete with hyperventilating and heart palpitations. Here's an example of the role perceptions play: Almost all of us initially react to public speaking with a full-blown stress response and high levels of adrenaline and cortisol. But after speaking a number of times, we realize it won't hurt us, and most of us don't perceive it as a threat anymore. A study showed that, after some experience with public speaking, 90 percent of people can handle it without elevated levels of stress hormones, but about 10 percent continue to find it incredibly stressful; their bodies respond every time as if a predator were chasing them (Kirschbaum et al. 1995).

If you don't perceive a situation as a threat, you'll handle it with less of an increase in adrenal activity—be it public speaking, being narrowly cut off on the freeway, or anything else. We've all had different life experiences that color how we respond to a given situation. Some of us have had a hard time of it and are generally "glass half empty" people, feeling concerned or fearful in a variety of situations. Others, for whatever reason, are of the "glass half full" variety.

Reactions can also vary in response to a sustained period of stressful experiences. If you've lost your job, your spouse has left you, or your teenage children are having problems, it tends to reduce your tolerance of stress. Your perception of a potentially stressful situation affects not only your initial adrenal response but also how well you recover from it afterward, once the danger is past, the infection has been contained, the surgery is over, or the speech has been given (Lazarus and Folkman 1984). For adrenal health, and overall health, it's important that elevated levels of cortisol and adrenaline return to normal after a stressful event, and that they do so relatively quickly. A slow return to normal levels has been linked to accelerated aging, as well as wear and tear on the brain that can lead to cognitive impairment (Sapolsky 1992).

The biological stress response is designed to be short-term and self-regulating, so if it's aroused too often or lasts too long, it can potentially affect your overall health and well-being. What happens if you're buffeted by nonstop stress and your levels of cortisol and adrenaline remain elevated? You might become mired in trouble at work, fights with your friends, difficulties at home, and so on. If your adrenals remain in a state of heightened alert and continue to produce adrenaline and cortisol, you're exposed to chronically elevated blood sugar, which raises insulin levels and can result in insulin resistance and type 2 diabetes. Your immune system stays on red alert and inflammatory activity becomes chronic. Fat and glucose are pulled from cells to deliver energy to muscles; in the long term, this can lead to the breakdown of tissues. This process can affect any organ or system in your body, causing inflammation and degenerative diseases.

And to top all this off, after an extended period of producing high levels of cortisol and adrenaline, your adrenals can start to tire to the point that they are unable to produce even sufficient levels of these hormones. This is a state known as *adrenal fatigue*. In either case—whether levels of stress hormones are too high or too low—your body can't adequately respond to stress and has a hard time maintaining balance, or homeostasis.

The trick to avoiding both types of imbalance is to make stress management part of your daily life. While there are many different techniques, the basic tenet is to learn to recognize what you can and cannot control. (I'll discuss methods of controlling your stress response in chapter 8.)

So how can you understand and resolve your own adrenal dysfunction? We need to begin at the beginning, with some simple definitions and descriptions of potential problems. Once you understand what's going on in your body and why, not only will the solutions make sense, your control of the information will help you to make the best decisions for your health.

HOW YOUR ADRENAL HORMONES WORK

You have two adrenal glands, each positioned above a kidney. Each adrenal gland is divided into two parts: the outer cortex and inner medulla.

The adrenal cortex produces cortisol, *aldosterone*, which helps maintain blood pressure and water and electrolyte balance, and various *androgens*—hormones that develop and maintain masculine characteristics.

The medulla makes adrenaline, which comes to your aid in times of stress in many ways: It increases your heart rate and the force of your heart's contractions. It narrows blood vessels and dilates air passages. It increases blood flow to your muscles and brain and causes smooth muscles to relax. The medulla also makes *noradrenaline*. Like adrenaline, it narrows blood vessels and increases blood pressure. Some telltale signs of increased noradrenaline are the feeling of your hair standing on end, gooseflesh, and dilated pupils. Watch children when they're engrossed in a scary movie and you'll see what I mean.

Adrenaline and cortisol are both secreted constantly in varying amounts to keep critical physiological systems operating in balance. They work hand in hand. Adrenaline is short acting. During a stress response, it starts things off by triggering a release of blood sugar stores from the liver and fatty acids from cells for quick energy. It spikes first, and then, when adrenaline levels start to drop, cortisol jumps in. Cortisol is long acting, with sustained momentum, so it builds up slowly and its levels take longer to return to normal. Cortisol helps keep energy levels replenished by supplying cells with amino acids as well as blood sugar and fatty acids. But if the elevated blood sugar and fats aren't consumed by a physical response, such as running or fighting, they'll accumulate. Over time, this leads to fat buildup, initially in the abdomen and the walls of blood vessels. An expanding waistline is a visible warning sign that fat is probably also building up in the blood vessels.

As seen in the following graph, the adrenaline production curve influences the cortisol production curve. With each spike in adrenaline, cortisol production increases, but at a slower pace. Because cortisol levels peak well after adrenaline levels, if another spike in adrenaline occurs relatively soon, there isn't time for cortisol to return to baseline levels, so cortisol levels continue to climb. And when you have high levels of cortisol flowing through your bloodstream, it takes longer to recover from an adrenaline surge. If you go from one stressor to the next without enough time to recover in between, your baseline level of cortisol eventually ramps up to a higher level, impairing your ability to recover from stress. This pattern of chronically elevated cortisol is associated with several conditions, including depression (Burke et al. 2005), weight gain, suppressed immune function, heart disease, and accelerated aging.

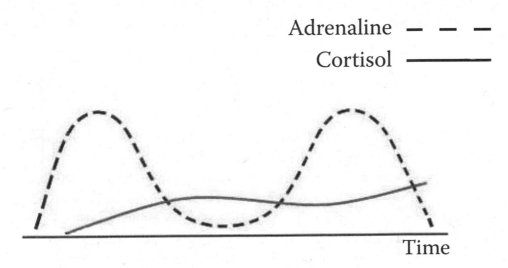

Relationship between cortisol and adrenaline production

When your cortisol and adrenaline levels are elevated, you'll initially feel good. Your mind will be sharp and focused. You'll have loads of energy. Your senses will become more acute. You'll have what's popularly known as an adrenaline rush. It's likely that you'll look good, too. It's only when your adrenals continue to produce high levels of these hormones that they will start to impact your health.

When your adrenaline level falls and the inevitable adrenaline crash hits, you may start to feel anxious and negative, maybe even irritable and depressed. It may seem paradoxical, but this is how the stress response works. You feel great when the adrenaline and cortisol are surging and feel bad when your body is relaxing afterward. This helps explain why we crave things that will keep these hormones elevated, from caffeine to extreme sports to overexercising. This also helps explain why it's so hard to fight these urges.

Adrenaline

So adrenaline delivers short-acting, emergency support in times of crisis. However, when adrenaline levels get too high and stay too high due to chronic stress, it can cause problems. In the beginning, there are no warning signs that your adrenaline level is chronically too high. In fact, you may feel so good that you convince yourself that your diet and lifestyle are perfect—even if you're eating only refined carbs or fast food and sleeping three hours a night. It isn't until this has gone on for a while and you've sustained significant damage to your metabolism that you'll begin to notice some signs of what's been going on beneath the surface.

You'll begin to look older than you should. Far more seriously, internally you may have started to develop degenerative conditions and, prematurely, diseases of aging. Chronic high levels of adrenaline can lead to heart problems, such as an irregular heartbeat, or damaged blood vessels, which make a heart attack or aneurysm more likely. Elevated adrenaline also causes blood to clot, increasing the risk of stroke.

Cortisol

Cortisol is in the category of hormones called glucocorticoids, which simply means hormones that affect the metabolism of carbohydrates and, to a lesser extent, fats and proteins. Cortisol keeps your body's reactions to stress in balance. It also has other vital functions, all related to the stress response: It increases blood sugar levels in the bloodstream. It directs the body to break down carbohydrates, fats, and proteins to produce energy. And it also regulates the immune system. Because cortisol has such a profound effect on a wide range of critical processes, cortisol levels must be tightly controlled by the body. Levels that are too high or too low can cause problems with all of these functions.

Cortisol has been enjoying a lot of notoriety recently. Misleading advertisements and television commercials have been demonizing it as the cause of weight gain. Products blocking its action, such as Relora, Relacore, and CortiSlim, are suddenly all the rage, being promoted for weight loss. While chronically high cortisol levels can result in abdominal weight gain, among other problems, the fact is, cortisol is necessary for life. Its roles in energy production, immune function, heart health, brain function, and gastrointestinal health are intrinsic to overall health.

Cortisol levels rise and fall over a twenty-four-hour period. Normally, they are highest in the first hour after waking. They drop sharply until 11 a.m. and then decline gradually throughout the rest of the day, hitting bottom between midnight and 2 a.m. This pattern can be affected when your adrenals are either too active or not active enough.

In addition to levels being too high or too low, the pattern of production can be disrupted in a variety of ways. You may have a high early morning peak but then your levels drop too quickly, leaving you exhausted by late morning or early afternoon. Or you may not produce the early morning peak, so you have a hard time getting started in the morning. You can even have a reversed pattern: levels of cortisol that are low in the morning and increase all day, peaking in the afternoon or evening. With this pattern, you'll feel tired all day but feel better in the late afternoon and best after dinner and into the evening. This can result in a lack of sleep, which has an overall effect of pushing levels of cortisol even higher (Laughlin and Barret-Connor 2000). Unfortunately, this is a common problem as we age.

An interesting study showed that light exposure in the early morning has a strong impact on the morning cortisol peak. For those who awoke to bright light, cortisol levels about half an hour after waking were 35 percent higher than for those who awoke during darkness (Frank, Scheer, and Buijs 1999). One easy way to help normalize your production pattern if your cortisol levels are low is to increase your exposure to sunlight during the day, especially in the early morning.

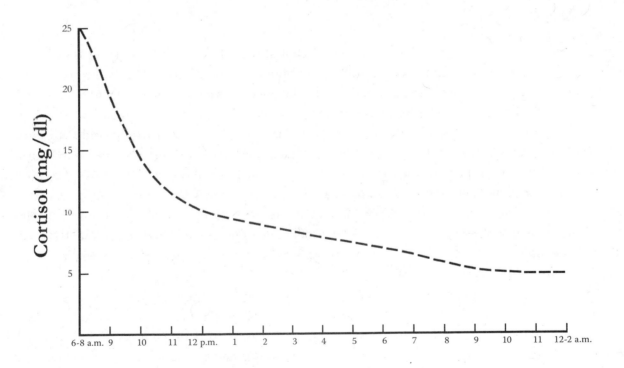

Normal cortisol production pattern

Source: Kathryn Simpson, *The Women's Guide to Thyroid Health* (Oakland, CA: New Harbinger Publications, 2009).

It's important that you understand your individual cortisol production pattern in order to best support or repair your adrenal function. In chapter 4 I'll explain the tests that your doctor can order to assess your cortisol production profile.

Aldosterone

Aldosterone is the most important adrenal hormone in a class called mineralocorticoids—hormones that regulate the body's balance of water and electrolytes, such as sodium and potassium, to control blood pressure, distribution of fluids, and other physiological functions.

Aldosterone acts on your sweat glands to reduce the loss of sodium when you sweat. It also acts on your taste buds to increase their sensitivity to the taste of salt. These are cleverly designed systems for keeping your sodium levels optimal. When levels of aldosterone are too high or too low, blood volume and blood pressure can also become too high or too low.

Pregnenolone

Your adrenals make several hormones out of cholesterol. The most important of these hormones is *pregnenolone*. Sometimes called the "mother of hormones," pregnenolone is the precursor, or building block, for many other hormones, including *progesterone* and *dehydroepiandrosterone* (DHEA), which in turn are converted into sex hormones such as estrogen and testosterone.

Pregnenolone is critical to brain function, particularly memory and learning, and the brain contains large amounts of it. Studies in animals show that low levels of pregnenolone impair memory and that supplemental pregnenolone can reverse this memory loss (Akwa and Baulieu 1999).

Studies also show that pregnenolone plays a role in nerve regeneration and repair. It dramatically improves spinal cord injuries and can potentially reverse paralysis when given immediately after an injury (Guth, Zhang, and Roberts 1994). Production of pregnenolone decreases with stress, aging, depression, hypothyroidism, and exposure to toxins. It can also be depleted when levels of other hormones, such as cortisol, are low, as it's used to replenish those supplies.

In the past, pregnenolone was used to treat arthritis, because the body converts it into cortisol when levels are low. Pregnenolone can also counter damage caused by excess cortisol and help to normalize cortisol levels. Among other things, excessive cortisol damages brain function, causing memory problems. Blocking this damage process may be one of the main reasons for the well-known memory-enhancing effects of pregnenolone. As with most other hormones, pregnenolone levels drop fairly drastically as we age—as much as 60 percent by the time we're seventy-five (Rothenberg and Becker 2007).

DHEA

DHEA is the most abundant hormone in your bloodstream, and it has important functions similar to those of cortisol. Evidence shows that it can improve immune function and stimulate white blood cell activity, helping you withstand viral and bacterial diseases (Jiang et al. 1998). DHEA has been proven to have potent anti-inflammatory properties, which fits with data showing that people with chronic inflammatory diseases often have lower levels of DHEA (Straub, Schölmerich, and Zietz 2000). In addition, DHEA supplementation has shown promise in treating autoimmune disorders like lupus and HIV infection, as well as a wide range of degenerative diseases (Bijlsma et al. 2002).

DHEA works in concert with other androgens to control masculine characteristics. Both men and women make DHEA in their adrenal glands. In adult males, the adrenals make much lower amounts of androgens than the testes do, but in females, the adrenals are a major source of androgens.

DHEA production generally starts to decline in our late twenties. Most seventy-year-olds have only 5 to 10 percent as much DHEA as twenty-eight-year-olds (Orentreich et al. 1984). However, DHEA levels can actually get too high when the adrenals first go into overdrive and start making too much adrenaline and cortisol.

Signs of too much DHEA are greasy hair and skin, acne, strong body odor, aggression, deepening of the voice, mood swings, and excessive growth of facial and body hair. In women, another sign is loss of menstrual cycles. One of the main causes of teenage acne in girls is elevated levels of DHEA and testosterone, creating an imbalance relative to estrogen.

ADRENALS AND THE ENDOCRINE SYSTEM

The adrenals aren't autonomous. Nothing in our bodies works in isolation; its interdependent systems nurture and support each other. When one system gets damaged or stops functioning correctly, a cascade of consequences flows throughout the body. Fortunately, the body has its own checks and balances. In addition, we can learn to read and understand these systems, which can help us manage them. Ultimately, this is the key to good health.

The adrenal glands are part of the *endocrine system*, a powerful group of organs and glands that includes the hypothalamus, pituitary, thyroid, parathyroid, thymus, adrenals, pancreas, reproductive glands (ovaries and testes), and pineal gland. Each of these glands produces hormones, which are released or stored depending on your body's needs. All of these glands are interrelated, and the adrenals play a particularly important role in this interplay.

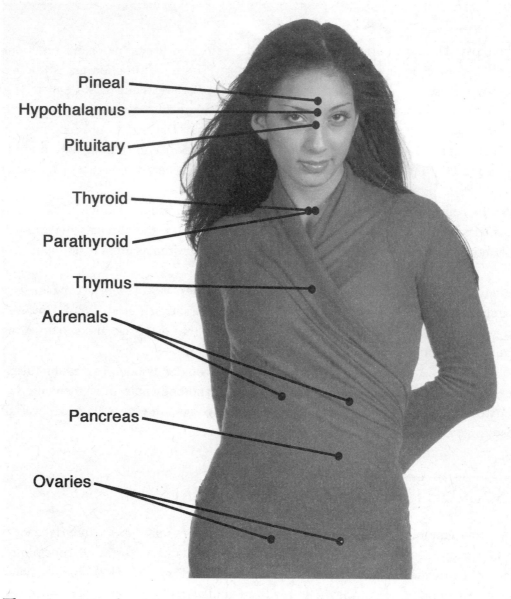

Pineal

Hypothalamus

Pituitary

Thyroid

Parathyroid

Thymus

Adrenals

Pancreas

Ovaries

The primary endocrine glands

Source: Kathryn Simpson, *The Women's Guide to Thyroid Health* (Oakland, CA: New Harbinger Publications, 2009).

These glands and their hormones communicate information throughout the endocrine system and to other parts of the body via the bloodstream. Together, they accomplish a huge number of essential activities, and all elements of the system are designed to work in a specific way. Adrenal hormones are programmed to interact with specific cells. After traveling through the bloodstream to reach target cells, they connect to cell receptors and deliver instructions that affect functions including energy production, blood pressure, cholesterol, and blood sugar levels.

The endocrine system's production and regulation of hormones begins in the hypothalamus, which is about the size of a small bean and located in the center of the brain. It sends instructions to the pituitary, which is situated just below it. The pituitary, in turn, tells all the other endocrine glands what to do. Any weakness in this chain of communication affects the entire system.

When you're faced with stress, your hypothalamus increases levels of corticotropin-releasing hormone (CRH) to send a message to your pituitary. This triggers your pituitary to secrete adrenocorticotropic hormone (ACTH) to instruct your adrenal glands to produce hormones, including cortisol, adrenaline, aldosterone, and DHEA. Once enough of these hormones are produced to help you cope with the stressful situation at hand, the message is passed back up the chain and production of regulatory hormones slows, reducing their levels.

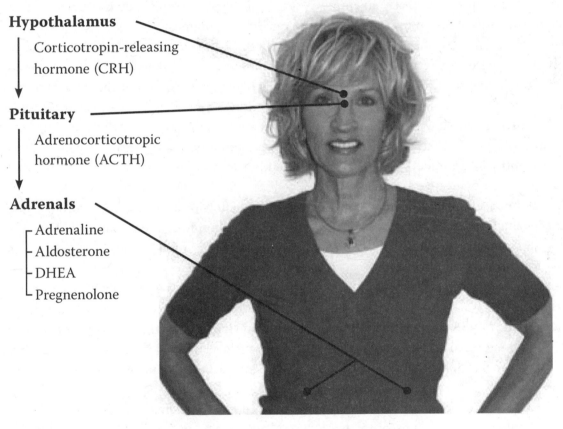

Hypothalamus

Corticotropin-releasing
hormone (CRH)

Pituitary

Adrenocorticotropic
hormone (ACTH)

Adrenals

Adrenaline
Aldosterone
DHEA
Pregnenolone

Adrenal stimulation pathway

ADRENALS, IMMUNE SYSTEM, AND INFLAMMATION

Your adrenal glands work hand in hand with your immune system (and nervous system) to manage inflammation in the body. Cortisol has the dual role of first helping your immune system launch an inflammatory response and then stopping the immune response when it's no longer needed. Inflammation occurs when your immune system is activated in response to injury, infection, or irritation. This is a good thing. The interconnected group of cells, tissues, and organs that comprise the immune system work together to repel the millions of bacteria, microbes, viruses, toxins, and parasites constantly trying to invade your body. This system is permanently on call to mobilize your defenses and fight off disease and the effects of injury.

When you catch a cold or pull a muscle, your immune system switches on and triggers a chain of events called an *inflammatory cascade*. The familiar signs of inflammation—swelling, pain, redness, and heat—signal that your immune system is working. Your body has alerted white blood cells to rush to the site to resolve infection or repair tissue damage.

Within this seemingly chaotic activity, there is a well-organized plan. Cortisol helps move immune cells to where they're needed. And after your immune system has done its job—resolving an infection, injury, or other threat—healthy adrenals release cortisol to put the brakes on the inflammatory cascade (McEwen et al. 1996). When everything works as it should, this process is an elegant balancing act. However, precise amounts of cortisol are needed to switch the immune system on and off. Levels that are too high suppress your immune system, leaving you with an increased susceptibility to infection. Levels that are too low lead to an increased susceptibility to inflammatory and autoimmune disorders.

Mild inflammation is inconvenient but livable: swelling joints or aches after a vigorous game of tennis, sneezing and itching after hugging your cat, streaming eyes when your neighbor cuts the grass, or a stomachache, swelling, or bloating after eating certain foods. But as we age, stress can take its toll and adrenal function can decrease, and the consequences of this impaired adrenal function can be acute. If you watch any television at all, you've seen the overwhelming number of advertisements for various anti-inflammatory drugs: statins for our arteries, nonsteroidal anti-inflammatory drugs (NSAIDs) and COX-2 inhibitors for our joints, Claritin and many others for allergy relief, and a long list of others. These drugs may provide superficial relief of symptoms, but they don't address what may be the underlying problem: increasing inflammation due to adrenal dysfunction.

When inflammation gets out of control, it can cause serious problems. It appears in different forms in different parts or systems of the body. It's called sinusitis in the sinuses and rhinitis in the nose—as most allergy sufferers know all too well. Then there's asthma, when inflammation is in your airways; arthritis, when inflammation is in your joints; and dermatitis, when inflammation affects your skin. In fact, the suffix "-itis" simply means "inflammation of."

Inflammation has also been implicated in high blood pressure (Chae et al. 2001), inflammatory bowel disease and irritable bowel syndrome (Dinan et al. 2006), depression (Raison, Capuron, and Miller 2006), high cholesterol (Alexander 1994), heart disease and autoimmune diseases like lupus, multiple sclerosis, and rheumatoid arthritis (Abou-Raya and Abou-Raya 2006), Alzheimer's disease (Vasto et al. 2008), and even cancer (Schleimer 2000).

THE ROLE OF THE ADRENALS IN CHRONIC HEALTH CONDITIONS

Consider your adrenal glands as "guardians at the gate" of stress. They're designed to secrete various hormones and inhibit others in response to stress. Their function involves constantly balancing levels of the two primary stress hormones: cortisol and adrenaline.

But if adrenaline and cortisol are constantly released by your adrenal glands or if their levels are poorly regulated, things start to break down. When cortisol levels are deficient, heightened immune activity can't be shut off once it's no longer needed. The off switch is broken. And when your immune system is always activated, your adrenals release even more cortisol in an attempt to counteract the situation and get things under control. This can ultimately suppress your immune system, resulting in chronic inflammation, which can lead to chronic disease.

History always gives us clues. If we look at our bodies in the context of how humans lived in past centuries, we see that many of the biochemical actions that are damaging us now were formerly necessary to survival. For example, before we had drugs like antibiotics, surviving acute infections or injuries required a robust inflammatory response that could mobilize the body's defenses and stave off bacterial and viral invaders. There were no other options.

Life is very different today. We live in a stressed-out civilization, and many of us feel overwhelmed by a seemingly inescapable environment of stress, from overwork, financial problems, relationship issues, and the responsibilities of parenting to sleepless nights and suboptimal diet and nutrition. On top of this, and perhaps even more importantly, we are exposed to environmental and chemical toxins that exist throughout the food chain, in our homes, and in the atmosphere.

All of these factors put tremendous stress on our bodily systems, causing our adrenals to produce stress-fighting hormones. Is it any wonder that our adrenal glands can get stuck on permanent overdrive, chronically producing stress hormones? And because the body is designed to produce these hormones sporadically, not continuously, the all-too-frequent result is that our adrenal glands wear out.

Over the past few decades, many scientists have come to believe that inflammation is at the root of most chronic health problems (Chiodini et al. 2007). In fact, an overloaded inflammatory process is found in most diseases (McEwen et al. 1996). A great deal of current medical research focuses on ways to treat the symptoms of damage caused by chronic inflammation.

In a recent study, researchers linked asthma and inflammation and found that men who took an aspirin (an anti-inflammatory drug) every other day were 22 percent less likely to develop asthma than those who did not (Barr et al. 2007). Researchers have even concluded that cancer is an out-of-control inflammatory condition (Rakoff-Nahoum 2006). The concept of cancer as an inflammatory disease isn't a new one; it's returning after a 150-year hiatus. German scientist Rudolph Virchow made this argument back in 1860.

With a steady stream of scientific research delivering insights into inflammation and its consequences, it's confusing that mainstream medicine has skipped over the fact that some of the hormones made in the adrenal glands do a remarkable job of reducing inflammation. Yet this is exactly what they're designed to do. If the adrenals are healthy, many aspects of chronic inflammation simply don't occur. So if we can address why the adrenals aren't functioning correctly and get them in good shape, the body can do what it's designed to do, with its natural rhythms and systems operating smoothly, efficiently, and successfully.

WHERE DOES THIS LEAVE US?

At this point you have a general understanding of the role that adrenal hormones play in various physiological functions and how they can be both beneficial and harmful. You also understand how the biological stress response, if triggered too often, can result in excessive production of adrenal hormones, with negative effects throughout the body, including an impaired immune system and inflammation.

Your ability to handle stress effectively is influenced by your underlying physical health, which is in turn influenced by genetic, lifestyle, and dietary factors. Your ability to cope with psychological stressors is also dependent on your perception of a situation. Whether you perceive a situation as a threat or not determines how you respond to it. Later in the book I'll offer strategies that can make you less subject to the harmful effects of stress. Chapter 7 will address diet, and chapter 8 will cover lifestyle issues and ways to modify your perception of and response to stress.

But first you need to determine whether your adrenals are making too many or too few hormones. The general pattern is excessive production of adrenal hormones for a sustained period of time, until the adrenals finally tire and then can't make sufficient amounts any longer. Both conditions—excessive and deficient stress hormones—can be detrimental to your health. The wonderful thing is, once you understand the signs and symptoms of these two conditions and what causes your adrenals to be either too active or not active enough, you can use this information to successfully optimize your health.

KEY POINTS

- The adrenal glands are responsible for responding to outside stress and restoring homeostasis, or balance, after a stress response.

- Your adrenal glands produce hormones that manage stress and control inflammation, including adrenaline, cortisol, aldosterone, pregnenolone, and DHEA.

- The production pattern for cortisol is just as critical as amounts. Your levels should be at their highest in the morning and decrease throughout the day.

- When stress is ongoing, cortisol levels become chronically elevated. This results in suppression of the immune system and sustained inflammation, which can lead to chronic disease.

- After producing excessive amounts of adrenal hormones in response to chronic stress, the adrenals can tire and produce inadequate amounts of these hormones, a condition known as adrenal fatigue.

CHAPTER 2

Adrenal Overdrive and Excessive Levels of Adrenal Hormones

Many of us live hectic lives filled with conflicting demands and challenges beyond our control: financial worries, relationship problems, workplace pressures, and more. You're probably all too familiar with scenarios like this: *Your project deadline is coming up. You start to panic. You don't have any of the data you need to put the final report together, let alone make coherent recommendations. Accounting isn't getting back to you, and even though marketing sent you a huge pile of stuff, you have no idea what the heck it all means. Your assistant said he heard that the CEO sent out an addendum, but he can't seem to find it. You spend hours looking for it in your e-mail files but keep forgetting what you're looking for. Everything seems to be closing in on you. Your blood pressure is rising, your pulse is racing, and you're anxious, yet this is just another "normal" day. In recent months, you haven't been able to sleep, you haven't even thought about sex, and your stomach has been in knots, yet you still manage to eat everything in sight. You can't fit into your pants, let alone think straight.*

You may feel angry, frustrated, tired, or sad. Part of you may know that something's wrong—you can feel it. If your blood pressure is rising, your heart is pounding, and you have emotional, digestive, and sleep disturbances, these are obvious indicators that your stress response has been triggered and your adrenals are flooding you with cortisol and adrenaline.

CAUSES OF EXCESSIVE PRODUCTION OF STRESS HORMONES

The scenario above is but one example of the ways day-to-day challenges can cause chronic stress. But there are also many stressors that can significantly raise cortisol and adrenaline levels even when you may not consciously feel stressed, making them hard to detect. Some of the most common stressors of this type are suboptimal diet and lifestyle, acute or chronic infections, hormone deficiencies and imbalances, environmental toxins, cortisol-like medications, and cortisol-producing tumors.

Diet and Lifestyle Stressors

Diet and lifestyle choices can trigger the stress response. If your diet is composed of lots of junk food and lacking an adequate balance of healthful fats, protein, and complex carbs, or if you consume a lot of caffeine or sugar, it can stress your body and cause your adrenals to make more cortisol and adrenaline than may be good for you. Following a calorie restricted diet or skipping meals also stresses the body and raises cortisol levels, as cortisol is produced in an effort to raise insufficient blood sugar levels (Bergendahl et al. 1996). In addition, smoking, drug use, or excessive alcohol consumption will stress the body and increase cortisol production.

In middle age, lack of sleep is a common trigger for the adrenals to make more stress hormones. When you don't sleep enough at night, your cortisol levels increase. In turn, increased cortisol causes you to reach for comfort foods high in refined or simple carbs and fat. Unfortunately, this raises your cortisol levels even higher, which can increase inflammatory activity, not to mention adding to that hard-to-lose spare tire around your middle.

Regular exercise is important to counter stress. It can help reduce elevated levels of stress hormones caused by the fight-or-flight reaction. But too much exercise can have some unintentional consequences. As we step up our cardio workouts or maybe add miles to our run, we also step up cortisol production. If the duration and intensity of your exercise regimen causes ongoing cortisol release, it will eventually result in all the negative effects of excessive cortisol production.

Infectious Stressors

Both acute and chronic, low-grade viral, fungal, parasitic, or bacterial infections are common catalysts for overproduction of cortisol (Sibbald et al. 1977). Cortisol is responsible for moving immune cells into place to fight and resolve infections. It's also responsible for turning the immune system off after its job is done. If an infection isn't resolved, the immune system remains activated and the adrenals continue to produce excess cortisol in an attempt to turn off the immune activity.

Hormone Deficiencies

Because the functions of the glands of the endocrine system are so closely intertwined, changes in one gland can affect other glands. For men and women alike, the body interprets declining levels of sex hormones as a stressor and pumps out cortisol to cope with the decline.

Men's production of testosterone typically begins to decrease when they are in their forties or older. Women's production of estrogen and progesterone begins to diminish when they are in their late thirties, forties, and fifties. Women's adrenals are further stressed when the adrenals become the primary source of sex hormones after menopause, as the ovaries reduce their production.

Low thyroid function, or hypothyroidism, also stresses the body and leads to an increase in adrenaline production.

Environmental Toxins

Every day we're exposed to hundreds, even thousands, of synthetic chemicals via the air we breathe, the food we eat, and contact with products that contain them. Because our bodies weren't designed to deal with these chemicals, the adrenals are called upon to produce cortisol to help launch and subsequently control an immune attack to contain their effects.

Many of these chemicals fall into a class known as xenoestrogens, because they mimic the female hormone estrogen. Xenoestrogens aren't rare, exotic chemicals. They're everywhere: in cosmetics, pesticides, nonstick pan coatings, and most plastics. When these plastics are used as packaging, or for baby bottles or water bottles, the xenoestrogens can leach into any food or liquid within. Excess estrogen can cause problems with cortisol synthesis, resulting in cortisol deficiency (Gell et al. 1998).

Medications and Tumors

Other factors that can cause excess exposure to cortisol are certain medications and tumors. Molecularly altered forms of cortisol, such as prednisone, prednisolone, and dexamethasone, mimic the action of cortisol. If taken in high enough doses, these drugs can have the same negative effects on the body as excess cortisol. In addition, oral contraceptives have been shown to increase cortisol levels (Katz et al. 1975).

A type of tumor known as an adenoma, located on the pituitary or adrenal glands, can excrete high levels of various adrenal hormones. It's unknown what causes these tumors, but they're rarely malignant. Women are more likely than men to develop them. Adenomas are responsible for 15 to 20 percent of cases of Cushing's disease, a condition of extremely high cortisol production (Bornstein, Stratakis, and Chrousos 1999).

EXERCISE: Are Your Adrenals Making Excessive Levels of Stress Hormones?

The first step in detecting and resolving elevated levels of stress hormones is to evaluate your symptoms. As you read through the following list of signs and symptoms of adrenal hormone overproduction, you may find it hard to believe that your adrenal glands can have such powerful effects throughout your body. But the truth of the matter is that optimum adrenal function plays an important role in maintaining health and quality of life as you age.

Filling out this questionnaire is one of the most important things you can do to regain or maintain good adrenal health. Your responses will give you and your doctor an understanding of your current adrenal status. If adrenal dysfunction is the cause of your symptoms, it's unlikely that you'll get any relief until this root cause has been resolved.

Read the statements below, decide on the level of severity or frequency of each sign or symptom, and circle the number that most accurately reflects how that statement applies to you. Notice that the last eleven symptoms have higher point values, as they're more significant. It's useful to fill out the questionnaire periodically so that you can assess your improvement, so you may want to make copies and leave this version blank.

0 = None or never   2 = Moderate or often

1 = Mild or occasionally   3 = Severe or always

At the bottom of each page, total up the points circled, then carry these totals forward to the end of the evaluation to get a total score.

0	1	2	3	I'm anxious and irritable; any kind of stress sets me off.
0	1	2	3	I get caught up in worries.
0	1	2	3	I'm more fearful than circumstances warrant.
0	1	2	3	I tend to feel guilty.
0	1	2	3	I bruise easily, and cuts are slow to heal.
0	1	2	3	I have elevated blood pressure.
0	1	2	3	I have high cholesterol with low HDL and elevated LDL.
0	1	2	3	I retain fluid.
0	1	2	3	I have food cravings and increased appetite.
0	1	2	3	I have hyperglycemia (high blood sugar).

Page total: _____

0	1	2	3	I have trouble sleeping.
0	1	2	3	I get mouth ulcers or cold sores.
0	1	2	3	I look older than my age.
0	1	2	3	I have memory and cognitive problems.
0	1	2	3	I'm losing muscle and I have muscle weakness.
0	1	2	3	I have thin skin.
0	1	2	3	I have stretch marks that aren't from being pregnant.
0	1	2	3	I have excessive hair growth.
0	1	2	3	I feel light-headed and dizzy, especially when I'm under stress.
0	1	2	3	I have an unusually fast or pounding heartbeat.
0	1	2	3	I tend to breathe quickly.
0	1	2	3	I sweat a lot even when I'm not exercising.
0	1	2	3	I'm drinking more alcohol than I should.
0	1	2	3	I tend to get infections.
0	1	2	3	I'm not interested in sex.
0	1	2	3	I need to urinate more often than seems normal.
0	1	2	3	I tend to feel agitated or nervous.
0	1	2	3	I get heartburn.
0	1	2	3	I have headaches.
0	1	2	3	I get very restless.
0	1	2	3	My face or skin flushes easily.
0	1	2	3	My hands tremble.
0	1	2	3	I tend to have trouble breathing.
0	1	2	3	I get blurry vision.

Page total: _____

0 1 2 3   I have thin extremities. My arms and legs seem to be wasting away.

0 1 2 3   I have a round, moon face.

0 1 2 3   I've gained weight around my stomach without changing my eating habits.

0 1 2 3   I've been diagnosed with osteopenia or osteoporosis.

For the rest of the questions, circle 0 for no or 20 for yes.

0 20   I have eczema, psoriasis, or urticaria.

0 20   I have bowel problems such as irritable bowel syndrome or inflammatory bowel disease.

0 20   I have panic attacks.

0 20   I have an ulcer.

0 20   I have gastroesophageal reflux.

0 20   I have insulin resistance.

0 20   I have metabolic syndrome, or syndrome X.

0 20   I have type 2 diabetes.

0 20   I've been diagnosed with depression.

0 20   I have chronic or severe allergies.

0 20   I have a chronic health condition or illness.

Page total: _____

Total Score: _____

Interpreting Your Results

If your total score is between 8 and 12, you're beginning to show signs of possible excess cortisol and adrenaline production. If your score is between 13 and 19, your condition is more serious. And if your score is over 19, you've probably experienced significantly elevated levels of cortisol and adrenaline on a chronic basis, which can affect your health and well-being. If your score is over 12 or if you have any of the last eleven serious symptoms, even if only to a mild degree or occasionally, make an appointment with your doctor to have your adrenal function evaluated.

Details on Items in the Symptom Evaluation

To understand your symptoms more fully, and to ensure that you can give your doctor full details, take some time to explore all of the symptoms you experience. In the table below, list all of the conditions or symptoms that you circled above and provide as much detail as you can about each one: When did it start? Do you still suffer from it? If not, how long did it last? What treatments have you tried, and what drugs have you taken? Also think about whether some sort of stress might have been a catalyst. For example, did the symptom start right after an accident, surgery, divorce, or some other major stressor? Take this information with you when you see your doctor for your adrenal evaluation so that you can provide a full picture of your adrenal health. If you need more room, copy the table or use a separate sheet of paper.

Symptom	Began/Duration	Treatments	Comments
Example: High blood pressure	46 yrs. of age 2 years, ongoing	None	My blood pressure has been elevated for the last two years. My doctor wants me to start taking blood pressure medication.
Example: Stomach weight gain	47 yrs. of age Last 2 years, ongoing	Many different types of diets: low-fat, low-carb, calorie restriction	Nothing I do, including exercise and diet, helps to reduce the fat around my middle.

Once you start taking steps to reduce your stress hormone levels, fill out the symptom questionnaire every three months until all of your symptoms are gone. You may be surprised at how quickly many of them resolve.

WHAT HAPPENS WHEN YOUR ADRENALS PRODUCE EXCESS HORMONES

When your adrenal stress response is triggered, your adrenals ramp up their production of hormones and shut down many normal bodily processes to focus on the perceived emergency: Immune function is suppressed, organ function and cell reproduction slow, sleep becomes more difficult, sex drive diminishes, damage to the heart and brain occur, and appetite actually increases. Increased levels of cortisol and adrenaline, as well as the adrenal hormones DHEA and aldosterone, can have the following effects on the body.

Effects of Excess Cortisol and Adrenaline

When levels of adrenaline and cortisol remain chronically elevated, your immune system is suppressed, your metabolism slows, and your body's rate of repair trickles to a crawl. On the other hand, blood pressure, weight, and incidence of heart disease increase, as do levels of cholesterol, triglycerides, blood sugar, and insulin (Whitworth et al. 2005). Aging accelerates, as does production of free radicals—those unstable molecules that damage cells and wreak other forms of physiological havoc (Lee, Ogle, and Sapolsky 2002).

Prolonged high levels of cortisol and adrenaline can also affect the feedback loop with the glands that regulate the adrenals: the hypothalamus and pituitary. The relationship between the adrenals, hypothalamus, and pituitary is called the hypothalamic-pituitary-adrenal axis (HPA axis). Chronic stimulation of this system by ongoing stress causes it to be overactive even when excess stress hormones should signal the pituitary and hypothalamus to put a damper on the stress response. This can damage cortisol receptors and the regulatory function of the HPA axis. It can also cause increased hyperreactivity to stress later in life. In fact, studies show that children who have had traumatic childhood experiences are more prone to anxiety and depression (Heim and Nemeroff 2001).

In the sections that follow, I'll discuss some of the physiological effects of long-term excessive levels of cortisol and adrenaline. Don't get discouraged by how extensive these effects are. All of these symptoms can be resolved by normalizing stress hormone levels and optimizing adrenal function.

ALTERED BODY COMPOSITION AND WEIGHT GAIN

Elevated cortisol can cause changes in body composition. It causes your body to store more calories as fat, especially around your stomach and the sides of your face (Rosmond, Dallman, and Björntorp 1998), and increases the breakdown, or catabolism, of muscles. The physical profile associated with chronic high cortisol is a rounded middle and face and underdeveloped arms and legs (Epel et al. 2000).

Excessive cortisol can also stimulate your appetite, causing overeating and cravings for sugary and high-calorie fatty foods that are too strong to fight. Another key issue in weight gain is the relationship between insulin, a hormone made in your pancreas, and cortisol. When your body is stressed, cortisol is released to raise levels of fat and glucose (blood sugar) in your bloodstream and thereby increase energy and muscle strength. The increased blood sugar stimulates increased insulin, which has the job of keeping blood sugar levels within a very narrow range. When insulin is released continually, your cells eventually become desensitized to it, and high levels of blood sugar and insulin build up in the blood. This can cause insulin resistance and eventually type 2 diabetes and syndrome X, sometimes called metabolic syndrome.

Syndrome X is a metabolic disorder characterized by a cluster of problems that appear together, including insulin resistance, obesity primarily in the middle of the body, high cholesterol (and usually high triglycerides), and high blood pressure (Vicennati et al. 2002).

IMMUNE DYSFUNCTION

The body needs just the right amount of cortisol for optimal immune functioning. When you have enough cortisol, but not too much, white blood cells are mobilized effectively to defend your body against injury and invaders. But when cortisol levels get too high, your immune response is suppressed and you become more vulnerable to disease.

HEART PROBLEMS

Adrenaline has a direct and immediate effect on your heart. It prepares your body for vigorous physical activity by way of increased heart rate, volume of blood pumped, and blood pressure. If ongoing stress keeps your heart in a constant state of heightened alert, high blood pressure (hypertension) can damage the lining of the blood vessels, causing inflammation and allowing circulating cholesterol to attach to the walls of blood vessels. The result is atherosclerosis and clogged blood vessels. If stress causes a sudden increase in blood pressure and this occurs too often in blood vessels with atherosclerosis, a heart attack can occur.

The stress response also causes your body to produce fibrinogen, a protein that causes blood to clot. Its purpose is to prevent you from bleeding to death if you're injured. However, chronic stress causes sustained elevation of this clotting effect, resulting in increased risk of blood clots, heart attack, or stroke.

IMPAIRED BRAIN FUNCTION

Cortisol influences memory and cognitive abilities. The same mechanisms that make your brain and memory function better when you're under mild short-term stress can damage it over the long haul. When stress occurs unabated, some neurons may atrophy, impairing memory, while other neurons may grow and enhance feelings of fear, causing anxiety (McEwen 2005).

Stress can also shrink the brain, destroy brain cells, and cause chronic inflammation, which can result in Alzheimer's disease (Stokes 1995). The brain is involved in shutting off the stress response, so damage to the brain due to excess cortisol can result in chronic cortisol production, a vicious cycle leading to further damage to the brain. Fortunately, studies show that this damage is potentially reversible if cortisol levels subside (McEwen 2002).

ENDOCRINE DYSFUNCTION

Elevated cortisol has many negative effects, but none more profound than its effect on the functioning of the endocrine system. It suppresses thyroid function, causes the pancreas to over-produce insulin, and suppresses ovarian function in women, inhibiting production of estrogen and progesterone (Chrousos, Torpy, and Gold 1998). This can cause women to stop ovulating and develop symptoms of low sex hormones that can mimic menopause. It also blocks testosterone's effects in men. Chronic high cortisol can also make the body resistant to thyroid hormones and sex hormones and unresponsive to cortisol and its effects (Chrousos, Detera-Wadleigh, and Karl 1993).

GASTROINTESTINAL PROBLEMS

When you encounter stress, your body turns its focus to energy production. This requires it to shut down functions that aren't related to this goal, including digestion and other gastrointestinal functions. However, diverting all your body's resources to resolving a crisis makes sense only for a very short time. When stress goes on longer than it should, it can lead to inflammation and tissue damage in the gastrointestinal tract, causing digestive problems and disorders such as inflammatory bowel disease and irritable bowel syndrome (Dinan et al. 2006).

WEAKENED BONES

Although we tend to think of the bones as fixed and unchanging, they are actually in a constant state of flux, a process called remodeling, in which bone cells are broken down (called resorption) and replaced. High cortisol affects the body's ability to maintain bone health because it suppresses production of sex hormones such as estrogens and androgens, which play a role in building and maintaining bone. It also causes bone to be resorbed more quickly (Chiodini et al. 2008). Lastly, elevated cortisol decreases absorption of minerals in the gut, reducing levels of calcium and magnesium, which are needed to build bone.

SLEEP PROBLEMS

Unhealthy high levels of nighttime cortisol are common when the adrenals are in overdrive. This can cause short sleep duration and increased sleep disturbances (Kumari et al. 2009). This is another vicious cycle, because sleep deprivation itself causes increased cortisol production. It also increases blood sugar levels, which can exacerbate insulin resistance.

ACCELERATED AGING

Chronically elevated cortisol can exhaust your body and cause premature aging. It allows increased damage by free radicals, which accelerates aging and the progression of neurodegenerative disease (Liu and Mori 1999). As mentioned in preceding sections, it can short-circuit your memory and concentration and cause brain damage and can also lead to bone loss and muscle wasting. Other effects that lead to premature aging include slow loss of fine motor coordination and impaired digestion and elimination.

The right amount of cortisol is also necessary for your thyroid to work efficiently. When thyroid function is impaired due to either high or low cortisol, symptoms of low thyroid function that resemble aging occur, including fatigue, dry skin and hair, premature graying, weight gain, hair loss, and cracked, brittle fingernails.

EMOTIONAL IMBALANCES

During a crisis, our sensory skills are enhanced and we become hypervigilant. This is great for dealing with concrete, short-term dangers, but if stress is chronic and we're in this state all the time, we jump at every sound and become anxious and irritable.

Chronic overproduction of cortisol can also lead to depression (Raber 1998). And both excess cortisol and adrenaline can cause anxiety disorders, panic attacks, phobias, and mood swings (Brown, Varghese, and McEwen 2004). Impulse control and emotional equanimity can also become impaired (Arnsten and Goldman-Rakic 1998).

⬆ *Helen's Story*

Helen, a CPA, was forty-six when she came to my clinic with insomnia, fatigue, chronic heartburn, weight gain, and elevated cholesterol, triglycerides, and blood pressure. She had a large stomach and a round face and was forty-five pounds over her optimum weight.

Her diet and lifestyle evaluation revealed quite a few problem areas: Her meals, generally eaten at her desk, consisted mainly of high-fat foods and refined carbs. She drank several glasses of wine every night and had five to six cups of coffee every morning. She'd gone through a divorce seven years earlier and admitted she'd let herself go. She didn't exercise, and she spent most of her time at work. She continued working after she got home, and slept, fitfully, an average of five to six hours a night. Her lab work showed several hormone imbalances: elevated cortisol throughout the day, elevated glucose and insulin levels, and low estrogen and progesterone.

Helen agreed to make significant diet and lifestyle changes. Because she was insulin resistant and on her way to type 2 diabetes, we encouraged her to take her diet seriously and adopt a diabetes diet. This meant switching from refined carbohydrates (sugars and processed grains) to complex carbs (whole grains, fresh produce, and legumes). It also meant achieving a better balance by reducing her overall carbohydrate intake and eating more high-quality fats and proteins. She started eating more fish, fresh vegetables, and fiber. She also started exercising regularly, doing aerobic exercise for thirty to forty-five minutes two days per week and resistance training for thirty minutes three other days.

To address the hormone imbalances, Helen started supplemental estrogen and progesterone. We also recommended several nutritional supplements to lower her cortisol levels and help normalize her sleep. Because of her elevated blood pressure, cortisol, and triglycerides, it was important for Helen to stop consuming caffeine and to reduce her alcohol consumption.

Within a month of changing her diet, Helen's heartburn disappeared and she started losing weight. After another three months, she was sleeping soundly for six to seven hours most nights and her energy level returned to normal. Helen's six-month lab tests showed normal cortisol, insulin, and glucose levels, and her estrogen level was three times higher than it had been. By this time she'd also lost twenty-five pounds (much of it in her stomach). Her new lifestyle had become second nature, and she was well on her way to her optimal weight. And perhaps best of all, she was noticeably calmer and happier, and her sense of well-being had returned.

Effects of Excess DHEA

Elevated DHEA levels cause an increase in masculine sexual characteristics. It's hard to tell when men have elevated DHEA levels because they already have these characteristics. But in women, DHEA is converted into testosterone, which can result in an imbalance with estrogen if testosterone levels get too high.

Effects include excess hair growth (hirsutism), deepening of the voice, enlargement of the genitalia, infertility, and loss of menstrual cycles (amenorrhea). In adolescent girls, elevated levels of DHEA can cause excess acne, adult body odor, and delayed puberty.

Effects of Excess Aldosterone

When your adrenals are in high gear, levels of aldosterone, the hormone that controls water and sodium balance, can also become elevated. This can lead to high blood pressure and low potassium levels, which may result in muscle cramps and weakness as well as numbness or tingling in your extremities (Benvenga et al. 2001). Studies show that up to 12 percent of people with high blood pressure may have excessive levels of aldosterone (Mulatero et al. 2004). High blood pressure is known to be a risk factor for heart disease, and animal studies confirm that excess aldosterone can cause heart disease (Catena et al. 2008).

WHERE DOES THIS LEAVE US?

You now you know what can trigger your adrenals to produce too many stress hormones and what can happen when they do. Elevated levels of stress hormones can disrupt nearly every system in your body. They can suppress your immune system, raise blood pressure, increase the risk of heart attack and stroke, cause infertility and hormone disruption, and accelerate the aging process. Long-term exposure to stress hormones can even affect your brain, making you more susceptible to anxiety, depression, and memory loss. Understanding how your body responds to stress so you can recognize the symptoms of elevated levels of stress hormones is an important first step.

You need to be able to read these symptoms and signs that tell you that your stress response has been triggered. Everyone's different, so you'll need to identify your own indicators. You may experience physical symptoms like racing heartbeat, shallow breathing, deep sighing, tension in your muscles, upset stomach, or headache. Or you may have psychological or emotional symptoms, such as depression, anxiety, hopelessness, frustration, anger, sadness, fear, or problems with concentration or memory.

When you experience any of these, or other signs and symptoms of adrenal hormone imbalance, it's time to get to the bottom of the situation, because sustained overproduction of adrenal hormones eventually leads to chronic underproduction of these hormones and adrenal fatigue. If you scored high on the questionnaire, it's important to reduce or manage stress and the stress hormones that accompany it. Learning coping skills is critical. Whether it involves seeking social support, taking deep breaths, counting to ten, or simply walking away when faced with a potential confrontation, it's important that you start changing the way you respond. See chapter 8 for more on stress reduction.

KEY POINTS

 Excess production of adrenaline and cortisol can be triggered by a myriad of stressors, ranging from psychological, hormonal, or nutritional factors to exposure to toxins and infectious agents.

 Elevated cortisol and adrenaline levels have profound physiological effects. They are involved in weight control, immune function, hormone and neurotransmitter balance, aging, sleep, overall well-being, and heart, brain, gastrointestinal, and bone health.

 After making too much cortisol for too long, your adrenals can eventually get tired and stop producing sufficient levels of cortisol—a condition known as adrenal fatigue.

CHAPTER 3

Adrenal Fatigue and Deficient Levels of Adrenal Hormones

What happens when we've been bombarded with too much stress for too long? Our adrenals get tired and stress hormone levels start to decline—and then all of the wonderful, health-enhancing things that they do for us don't happen: Our energy reserves aren't replenished, our memory isn't enhanced, and our immune system isn't supported and controlled.

The beautiful, interconnected system that protects our bodies starts to weaken as low adrenal function has ripple effects on other systems. The immune system, normally contained by cortisol, becomes hyperactive, allowing inflammatory activity to increase and potentially causing conditions like allergies or asthma—or, if the situation goes on too long, causing autoimmune disorders like arthritis, lupus, and MS (Munck, Guyre, and Holbrook 1984).

Our stress response is genetically designed to protect us from danger, but the inevitable wear and tear on our adrenals from ongoing physical and psychological stress, compounded by diet and lifestyle challenges, can take a huge toll and result in adrenal fatigue. This is the point at which the demands of stress outweigh our resilience, and our adrenals start to lose their battle to maintain equilibrium, or homeostasis.

If the following scenario sounds familiar, you could be suffering from adrenal fatigue: *You drag yourself out of bed after another restless night with four or five hours of sleep. You stumble to the bathroom but have to sit on the edge of the tub because you feel dizzy and weak. Breakfast is donuts and several cups of coffee—it seems that you're craving sweets and stimulants all the time now. You get to work on time, although you can't really remember driving there. A coworker makes a comment about a project that you're late on, and before you can stop yourself, you lose your temper and launch into a tirade. Afterward, you feel shaky and weak, and it takes you a long time to calm down. It seems that everyone around you is incredibly annoying recently. By lunch you're ready to lie down for a nap, and you need more sugar or caffeine to make it through the rest of the day. Your fatigue seems to get a bit better after dinner and you can finally get things done, but once again you can't fall asleep until early morning.*

CAUSES OF ADRENAL FATIGUE

Stress is the most common cause of adrenal fatigue. There are several other catalysts for adrenal fatigue, as well, including hypothyroidism, congenital or hereditary factors, pituitary or hypothalamus dysfunction, adrenal antibodies, medications that suppress adrenal function, and vitamin D deficiency.

Stress

Adrenal fatigue can be caused by too much physical or emotional stress for too long. This means continual or extreme exposure to any of the stressors discussed in chapter 1: emotional, dietary, lifestyle, hormonal, environmental, or infectious. In fact, tuberculosis was one of the main causes of adrenal gland destruction in the past. Today, tuberculosis doesn't pose a big threat in the United States, but other acute or chronic infections, including respiratory infections like bronchitis, influenza, and pneumonia, can also deplete your adrenals. Acute or severe short-term stress can also damage the adrenals. Studies have linked many types of traumatic stress exposure, including abuse and neglect in childhood and post-traumatic stress disorder (PTSD), to low levels of cortisol (Boscarino 2004).

Like any other part of your body, your adrenal glands can get worn out. Just as playing too much tennis can tire your arm muscles, too much hormone production can tire the adrenals. Like a muscle, they get larger to increase output, but after they tire and can't keep up this production level, they start to shrink and can eventually atrophy.

Hypothyroidism

When the thyroid is underactive, a condition known as hypothyroidism, it doesn't adequately stimulate the adrenal glands to produce cortisol and other adrenal hormones. The end result can be adrenal fatigue. This is explained in detail in chapter 6, Understanding the Relationship Between the Adrenals and the Thyroid.

Congenital or Genetic Factors

Adrenal insufficiency can be caused by *congenital* factors (meaning present at birth but not necessarily genetic) or *genetic*, or hereditary, factors. Among the causes of congenital problems are nutritional deficiencies and toxins like heavy metals being passed from mother to child during pregnancy.

If your mother or father had compromised adrenal function when you were conceived, your embryonic development may have been influenced by this weakness. Think of the stressful situations many of our parents went through before we were born: the Great Depression, wars, or other traumatic events. Clinical studies have shown that wartime trauma experienced by a mother can lower adrenal function and cortisol levels in any children born to her after that time (Yehuda et al. 2007). How many of us had parents who served in or suffered through World War II, the Korean War, or another conflict? This influence on children's adrenal function may offer an explanation for why so many of us have adrenal fatigue.

Mild congenital adrenal hyperplasia is a condition caused by deficiencies in the adrenal enzymes that are used to synthesize cortisol. It leads to deficiencies of cortisol, and sometimes aldosterone, and excess production of androgens. In women, this condition can cause lack of ovulation, irregular menstrual cycles, infertility, and excessive hair growth. In both genders it can lead to short stature, strong body odor, and acne. It's estimated that 8 percent of women with polycystic ovary syndrome have congenital adrenal hyperplasia (Sahin and Kelestimur 1997).

In the past, adrenal hyperplasia was generally considered a rare inherited disorder with severe, life-threatening symptoms, but doctors who specialize in adrenal health have found that mild congenital adrenal hyperplasia is quite common. This frequently overlooked condition affects 1 in 100 to 1,000 people in the United States and occurs much more frequently in Hispanic, Slavic, and Italian populations, as well as Ashkenazi Jews (Deaton, Glorioso, and McLean 1999).

Problems with the Pituitary or Hypothalamus

Malfunction of either of the glands that help regulate the adrenals—the hypothalamus and the pituitary—can cause your adrenals to lose function. When these regulatory glands don't send the right signals, your adrenals won't make enough cortisol and other hormones. This can be a congenital problem, or it may be caused by injury or a viral or bacterial infection (Alevritis et al. 2003). This condition is called *secondary adrenal insufficiency*, as opposed to *primary adrenal insufficiency*, which occurs when the adrenal glands themselves malfunction.

Adrenal Antibodies

Your immune system can make antibodies that attack and destroy your adrenal glands instead of their usual targets, such as bacteria and viruses. The reasons for this condition are unknown. Adrenal antibodies are generally responsible for Addison's disease, which afflicted John F. Kennedy. This condition, which results in dangerously low levels of cortisol and sometimes aldosterone, occurs in about 1 in 100,000 people (Martorell, Roep, and Smit 2002).

Synthetic Cortisol-Like Drugs

Using drugs with longer-acting synthetic forms of cortisol, such as prednisone and prednisolone, for an extended period can suppress adrenal function. Your pituitary gland can't tell the difference between natural cortisol and these synthetic medications. It thinks you have enough cortisol and stops producing ACTH, so your adrenals aren't stimulated to make cortisol.

If you use these drugs for an extended period and then stop taking them abruptly, your adrenals won't be able to pick up cortisol production immediately. The result looks just the same as adrenal fatigue, and it can take months for your adrenal function to return to normal. Because of this, use the lowest possible doses of these drugs, and when you stop using them, cut the dosage back slowly. You'll need to work with your health practitioner on this.

Vitamin D Deficiency

Though we refer to it as a vitamin, vitamin D is actually an important hormone. While vitamin D deficiency doesn't generally cause adrenal fatigue, it can contribute to inadequate adrenal function. Vitamin D increases expression of the enzyme necessary for the production of adrenaline and noradrenaline (Puchacz et al. 1996).

With the aid of sunlight, your skin, kidneys, and liver produce vitamin D from cholesterol. Unfortunately, sun exposure alone can't produce enough vitamin D. You must also be able to manufacture it in your organs—but many of us over forty don't make enough of it to meet our needs.

Factors that decrease vitamin D levels include aging, use of sunscreens, low-cholesterol diets, and use of statin drugs, which decrease cholesterol production. Physical or emotional stress depletes vitamin D, as cortisol is also made from cholesterol, and when the body has to choose between making cortisol or vitamin D, it chooses cortisol to meet what it perceives as more immediate survival needs.

According to survey data, many of us are deficient in vitamin D. Doctors specializing in hormones recommend maintaining a vitamin D level of at least 55 nanograms per milliliter (ng/ml). Studies show that between 1988 and 1994, 45 percent of people in the United States had blood levels of at least 30 ng/ml of vitamin D, but just a decade later, only 23 percent did (Yetley 2008). Another study found that 9 percent of the U.S. population aged one to twenty-one were deficient in vitamin D, with levels under 15 ng/ml, and that 61 percent (50.8 million) had levels between 15 and 29 ng/ml (Reis et al. 2009). Yet another study found that in people over age ninety, high levels of vitamin D and normal thyroid function were the strongest indicators of longevity and health (Mariani et al. 1999).

EXERCISE: Do You Have Adrenal Fatigue?

A complete list of your current symptoms is necessary for your doctor to accurately diagnose and treat adrenal fatigue. You probably haven't gone to the same doctor your whole life, so you're the only person who has all the necessary historical information. Doctors generally have to try to piece together what's going on, and they're only as good as the information you give them. Take the information you compile in this evaluation with you when you go for your appointment.

The following questionnaire will help you determine whether you may be suffering from low adrenal hormone production and adrenal fatigue. You'll notice that a few of the symptoms of adrenal fatigue are similar to those of elevated levels of stress hormones. This is because many of the symptoms of excess cortisol remain even after your adrenals are making too little cortisol. With some symptoms, like inflammatory bowel disease, the inflammatory process, which began when the immune system was suppressed, can't be turned off because of insufficient levels of cortisol. Or with weight gain, for example, weight loss can't occur when cortisol levels are too low.

If you've checked off a number of symptoms on both questionnaires, you may wonder if there's any way to use this information to determine which is more likely to be your problem: too many adrenal hormones or too few. There is. Compare the number of symptoms you checked in each assessment. If most of your symptoms are on the list below, not in chapter 2, you probably had a period of adrenal hormone overproduction that led to adrenal fatigue and insufficient levels of these hormones.

Read the statements below, decide on the level of severity or frequency of each sign or symptom, and circle the number that most accurately reflects how that statement applies to you. Notice that the last ten symptoms have higher point values, as they're more significant. It's useful to fill out the questionnaire periodically so that you can assess your improvement, so you may want to make copies and leave this version blank.

0 = None or never

1 = Mild or occasionally

2 = Moderate or often

3 = Severe or always

At the bottom of each page, total up the points circled, then carry these totals forward to the end of the evaluation to get a total score.

0   1   2   3   I feel tired or fatigued.

0   1   2   3   My lips and face are pale.

0   1   2   3   I have cold sweats.

0   1   2   3   I tend to get anxious.

0   1   2   3   I get pain in my muscles and/or joints, including my neck, back, or groin.

0   1   2   3   I'm sensitive to heat.

0   1   2   3   I have dark circles under my eyes.

0   1   2   3   I drink more alcohol than I used to.

0   1   2   3   The lymph glands in my neck are swollen, painful, or tender.

0   1   2   3   I feel like I'm shivering or shaking inside.

0   1   2   3   I get moody and irritable.

0   1   2   3   I feel tired in the morning. I don't feel refreshed no matter how much sleep I've had.

0   1   2   3   I'm sensitive to environmental scents like perfume, chemicals, or air pollution.

0   1   2   3   I get respiratory infections that are hard to get rid of.

0   1   2   3   I have thin or scaly skin.

0   1   2   3   I seem to get sick more than other people and have a hard time bouncing back.

0   1   2   3   My cheeks or eyes look sunken.

0   1   2   3   I have the most energy after dinner and in the evening.

0   1   2   3   I have to drink coffee or other caffeinated beverages to keep going.

0   1   2   3   I feel like I'm going to faint.

0   1   2   3   I have abdominal pain, gas, or an upset stomach.

0   1   2   3   I panic and forget people's names.

0   1   2   3   I feel isolated and avoid social engagements.

0   1   2   3   Light bothers my eyes, and I'm uncomfortable when I don't wear sunglasses.

0   1   2   3   I can't take deep breaths.

0   1   2   3   My palms are cold and clammy.

0   1   2   3   I crave sweets and chocolate.

Page total: _____

0	1	2	3	I crave salty foods.
0	1	2	3	I'm sensitive to color, sound, and smells.
0	1	2	3	I smoke cigarettes more than I used to.
0	1	2	3	I get hissing sounds in my ears.
0	1	2	3	I get angry easily, and it takes me a long time to recover afterward.
0	1	2	3	I have brain fog and can't concentrate,
0	1	2	3	I don't like to talk to people or do any of the things I used to enjoy.
0	1	2	3	I have signs of dehydration, such as sharp wrinkles, and my skin forms stiff folds when I pinch it.
0	1	2	3	I have a hard time making sense out of things and feel like I'm not as smart as I used to be.
0	1	2	3	I have very little body hair.
0	1	2	3	I'm losing weight in my face; it's gotten thin.
0	1	2	3	I wake up at night and have a hard time breathing.
0	1	2	3	I have heart palpitations, particularly when I lie down at night.
0	1	2	3	My muscles are weak and stiff.
0	1	2	3	I have darker pigmentation at my temples, and I have red palms or fingertips.
0	1	2	3	I can't lose the weight I've gained around my waist.
0	1	2	3	I feel better when I'm lying down.
0	1	2	3	I have thin muscles no matter how much exercise I get.
0	1	2	3	I have crowded lower teeth and a high palatal arch (the roof of the mouth).
0	1	2	3	I have pain and tenderness in my mid back area when pressure is applied.
0	1	2	3	I have either very frequent urination in small amounts or infrequent in large amounts.
0	1	2	3	I can't fall asleep; I lie awake for hours.
0	1	2	3	I have a hard time exercising and get tired easily.
0	1	2	3	I have a weak or slow pulse.
0	1	2	3	I crave refined carbohydrates, like white bread and pasta.
0	1	2	3	My memory is getting bad.

Page total: _____

0   1   2   3   I don't sweat much.

0   1   2   3   My ankles and/or fingers swell.

0   1   2   3   I don't have much of an appetite anymore.

0   1   2   3   I tend to get respiratory infections.

0   1   2   3   I get PMS (premenstrual syndrome).

0   1   2   3   I startle easily at loud sounds.

0   1   2   3   Eating sweets makes me feel better.

0   1   2   3   I take things too seriously and get defensive easily.

0   1   2   3   When standing from sitting or from lying down, I feel light-headed or dizzy.

0   1   2   3   I have chronic infections like urinary tract infections or frequent colds, and have a hard time getting over them.

For the rest of the questions, circle 0 for no or the number on the right for yes.

0   5   When standing from sitting or from lying down, I feel light-headed or dizzy.

0   5   I feel ill or shaken after stressful events; I feel like I can't handle stress.

0   10   I have low blood pressure, and it drops further when I go from sitting to standing.

0   10   I have hypoglycemia.

0   20   I have asthma.

0   20   I have arthritis.

0   20   My skin has gotten darker as if I have a tan, but I haven't been in the sun.

0   20   I have low thyroid function, but when I tried thyroid medication it didn't work or I felt worse.

0   20   I have an autoimmune disease.

0   20   I have fibromyalgia.

Total Score: _____

Interpreting Your Results

If your total score is between 10 and 19, you may be in the early stage of adrenal fatigue. If your score is between 20 and 30, you're probably suffering from adrenal fatigue, which may be starting to affect the function of other hormones as well. If you scored over 30, your adrenal fatigue is potentially severe.

If your score is 10 or higher, it's important to do the easy home tests recommended in chapter 4, which will help you get a better picture of your adrenal health. Then schedule an appointment with your doctor for a thorough adrenal evaluation, including testing blood levels of adrenal hormones (also explained in chapter 4). Because thyroid dysfunction is often involved in adrenal problems, go ahead and fill out the thyroid evaluation in chapter 6 so you can take that information to your appointment as well.

Details on Items in the Adrenal Symptom Evaluation

To understand your symptoms more fully, and to ensure that you can give your doctor full details, take some time to explore all of the symptoms you experience. As in chapter 2, note any of the symptoms you circled above, and provide as much detail as you can about each one. If you need more room, copy the table or use a separate sheet of paper.

Symptom	Began/Duration	Treatments	Comments
Example: Chronic fatigue	45 yrs. of age 3 years; still have it.	Drink caffeine	The fatigue started after I had my last child at 41.

Once you start taking steps to repair your adrenal function, fill out the symptom questionnaire every three months until all of your symptoms are gone. You may be surprised at how quickly many of them resolve.

WHAT HAPPENS WHEN YOUR ADRENALS DON'T PRODUCE ENOUGH HORMONES

As your adrenal glands start to tire, they begin to shrink and hormone production dwindles. This is generally a long, slow process. Because it comes on gradually, sometimes it's not easy to figure out what's going on right away. You may start feeling a bit more tired or weak than usual. Or you may start having a hard time getting to sleep or notice that you're uncomfortable in bright sunlight without sunglasses. In the initial phase of adrenal fatigue, your body produces enough cortisol for most of your everyday activities but not enough to handle stressful situations.

If your adrenal function continues to decline, you may notice that even minor stress or conflicts can leave you feeling shaken or ill. Mild illnesses like colds and flu become more debilitating and seem to linger forever. You become ultrasensitive to environmental factors like bright lights, changes in temperature, and all kinds of smells. You can continue like this for an indefinite period. But if you then experience a serious trauma like a major injury, illness, or emotional setback, such as a divorce or job loss, your adrenal function and cortisol production will be further impaired, resulting in adrenal fatigue.

⬅ *My Story*

I had no idea I was on the road to adrenal fatigue. I was always energetic, working long hours as an executive in biotech and technology companies for more than twenty years. I left for work by 6:30 a.m. and seldom ate breakfast—I wasn't hungry, so why waste the time? I grabbed a snack at the office for lunch, usually a salad or a granola bar. I had dinner late, after a ten- to twelve-hour workday, and ate what we all thought was healthy back then: meals high in carbohydrates and low in fat. Unfortunately, I ate refined carbs instead of complex and cut out all fats and animal protein (because of the saturated fat). And, of course, I thought I didn't have time to exercise.

In my late thirties I took a stressful job as CEO of a startup company (and had my second and third sons) and started getting disturbing symptoms. The first was fatigue. Although I'd always had lots of energy, it was all I could do to get through the day. I hadn't been much of a coffee drinker before, but now I found I needed a double cappuccino to get me through the morning, then iced tea at lunch and coffee in the afternoon to get me through the rest of the day.

Then my hands went numb. It started in my right hand and spread to my left a couple of months later. Over the next few years, I developed chronic back pain and had infrequent but painful bouts of gastrointestinal reflux and gallbladder attacks. I became a bit unsteady on my feet and had to give up shoes with heels. I had a hard time falling asleep, which exacerbated my chronic fatigue. I tried all sorts of diets, even macrobiotic. But because I didn't understand the basic concept of what a healthy diet is—a balance of complex carbohydrates, high-quality protein, and healthy fats at every meal—I wasn't getting the nutrition I needed.

I got progressively more debilitated and was ultimately given a diagnosis of multiple sclerosis. My doctors basically told me to accept my fate and think about eventually getting a wheelchair. This stopped me in my tracks and forced me to dedicate myself full-time to figuring out what was going on in my body.

Years of research later, and after some trial and error, I emerged from a limited life with disabling symptoms into restored health. The key to my recovery lay in rebuilding my adrenal glands through good nutrition, balanced diet, daily exercise, eight hours of sleep a night, and supplementing with bioidentical *cortisol (meaning cortisol in exactly the same molecular form as naturally occurs in the body). I discovered that I also had deficiencies of thyroid hormones, estrogen, and progesterone, and resolved those by supplementing with bioidentical forms, as well. The difference in my health and well-being ever since has been incredible. I have robust adrenal health and no longer have any symptoms of adrenal fatigue—or multiple sclerosis!*

Effects of Deficient Cortisol and Adrenaline

Adrenal fatigue not only causes your adrenals to produce lower levels of cortisol and adrenaline, it can also cause disruptions in the circadian rhythm of cortisol production. This results in lower levels of cortisol in the morning, making it harder to start your day, and increased levels of cortisol at night, which can cause sleep problems.

Adrenal fatigue often causes few symptoms until your cortisol and other adrenal hormone levels have dropped appreciably. Symptoms of adrenal fatigue are both numerous and diverse and include fatigue, low blood sugar, low blood pressure on standing, and emotional problems. Over time, other symptoms develop, including weight loss (particularly on the sides of the face), increased skin pigmentation, and decreased underarm and genital hair (caused by low production of androgens by the adrenals). The following sections examine some of the effects of adrenal fatigue.

LOWERED ENERGY LEVELS

One of the scourges of modern life is the constant exhaustion many of us feel. We write it off as being too busy, working full-time, raising kids, and so on. But the truth is that these things don't tend to cause the kind of chronic exhaustion that forces you to lie down in the afternoon or make excuses to get out of evening activities.

When your adrenals are fatigued, you'll feel chronically tired. Cortisol plays a key role in balancing blood sugar, so it helps your body manage your daily ebbs and flows of energy. It also helps release energy from your body's fat stores for use by tissues and muscles.

ONGOING WEIGHT GAIN

As mentioned, years of high cortisol levels can cause your body to accumulate abdominal fat. Then, when your adrenal glands start to tire and your cortisol levels get too low, weight loss may become exceedingly difficult, since you need a certain amount of cortisol to burn fat weight off.

Low cortisol also causes blood sugar levels to decrease. As a result, you'll crave foods like sugar, refined carbs, alcohol, and stimulants. All can help raise blood sugar levels, but they can also quickly lead to additional weight gain (Mendelson, Ogata, and Mello 1971).

ACCELERATED AGING

Low cortisol levels can lead to accelerated aging, as this adrenal hormone is needed for nearly all dynamic processes in the body: building muscle and fat, synthesizing proteins, optimal immune function, and more—basically all those things that keep us young and energetic. Low cortisol levels can cause exhaustion, muscle loss, and muscle and joint weakness and pain and cause you to give up the activities of youth that can help keep you in good shape, such as sports and other types of exercise (D. Wilson et al. 1998).

IMPAIRED IMMUNE FUNCTION

Cortisol works hand in hand with your immune system to both mobilize immune activity and stop it when it's no longer needed. When cortisol is deficient, your immune system can't mount an optimal immune attack, and then it can't stop the immune activity, leading to an out-of-control immune response. Allergies are a good example of this lack of braking ability. Without controls, the immune system starts to react to substances that it normally takes in stride, like pollen and dander in the air and gluten and dairy in the diet. Taken a step further, this situation can result in autoimmune disease, where the body attacks itself.

Suboptimal immune activity due to low levels of cortisol leaves your body prey to recurrent infections, especially respiratory infections such as pneumonia (Gotoh et al. 2008). And, in a vicious cycle, even a minor tooth infection or an undetected intestinal infection with *Heliobacter pylori* (which causes ulcers) can be a constant source of inflammatory activity and take a big toll on your adrenals (Loesche 1994). If you have signs of a localized infection such as pain, swelling, or other discomfort, whether in your mouth, urinary tract, prostate, or elsewhere, get it checked out and treated. It can help take some of the burden off your adrenals, and when your adrenal health improves, it will be much harder for infections to take hold.

Asthma has also been linked to deficient adrenal activity and low adrenaline production. One clinical study showed that asthma sufferers had significantly lower levels of adrenaline than those without asthma (Mathé 1971). In another study, adrenaline levels in asthmatic patients didn't increase in times of stress, when they would normally spike, indicating adrenal dysfunction (Feng and Hu 2005).

DISRUPTED NEUROTRANSMITTER FUNCTION

Some neurotransmitters, including dopamine, are synthesized in the adrenal glands. In fact, among their many functions, adrenaline and noradrenaline also act as neurotransmitters. Adrenal fatigue can cause deficiencies in these important substances, with possible neurological consequences such as Parkinson's disease. In fact, grafting of dopamine-producing adrenal tissue into the brain has been employed as a neurosurgical approach to dopamine replacement therapy in Parkinson's disease (Kish, Shannak, and Hornykiewicz 1988).

SLEEP PROBLEMS

Cortisol has been shown to play an important role in regulating sleep. Abnormally low cortisol causes difficulty in falling asleep. It also leads to decreased time spent in REM (rapid eye movement) sleep and fewer REM sleep episodes (García-Borreguero et al. 2000). It's been suggested, but not conclusively proven, that REM sleep improves memory recall. Although benefits of REM sleep are still somewhat unclear, it obviously plays a fundamental role in sleep.

BEHAVIORAL CHANGES

Deficient cortisol results in behavior changes that may include increased anger and even psychopathic tendencies (Honk et al. 2003). It's also associated with aggression, depressed mood, and lack of impulse control and emotion regulation (Stansbury and Gunnar 1994). Studies have shown that low cortisol levels caused by an underfunctioning HPA axis may be the cause of attention deficit/hyperactivity disorder (ADHD) and oppositional defiant disorder (ODD) in adolescents (Kariyawasam, Zaw, and Handley 2002).

Effects of Deficient DHEA

When the adrenals become fatigued, DHEA production slows alongside cortisol production. The relationship between cortisol and DHEA levels is a valuable indicator of adrenal status. After an extended period of elevated levels of adrenal hormones, DHEA levels usually drop before cortisol. Much less commonly, DHEA remains high and cortisol drops first.

The ratio of cortisol to DHEA increases significantly as we age and is even higher in people with dementia. DHEA is important in helping the brain resist changes brought on by stress. When DHEA levels decline relative to cortisol, this may contribute to the onset and progression of the neurodegenerative diseases of aging (Ferrari et al. 2001).

In addition, this imbalance has been linked to degenerative conditions like cognitive impairment (Kalmijn et al. 1998), rheumatoid arthritis (Masi et al. 1998), and inflammatory bowel disease (Straub et al. 1998). Other studies link low DHEA levels to various cancers, inflammatory disease, type 2 diabetes, and cardiovascular disorders (Shealy 1995). In many of these studies, DHEA was shown to have decreased before the onset of disease symptoms, suggesting that low levels of DHEA are the cause, not the result, of the illness (Hinson and Raven 1999).

Effects of Deficient Aldosterone

With adrenal fatigue, levels of aldosterone can also become deficient. This results in less sodium being retained. So if you find yourself craving chips, nuts, or anything salty, you may have low levels of aldosterone. Aldosterone deficiency can also cause low blood pressure and rapid pulse rate, heart palpitations, and dizziness or light-headedness upon standing. Low aldosterone also increases potassium levels in the body and affects thirst and urination, sometimes causing people to urinate as many as fifteen to twenty times a day and drink a huge amount of water.

Signs of low aldosterone are water retention (swollen hands and feet) and, less often, a reddish, swollen face. Although the common way to reduce swelling is to take diuretics, with an aldosterone deficiency this can further compound dehydration and electrolyte imbalances and make you feel worse.

🍃 Lauren's Story

Lauren, a single parent with a fourteen-year-old daughter and a twelve-year-old son, was forty-four when she came to my clinic. She'd been divorced three years earlier, and within a year had started to suffer from chronic fatigue. More recently, she'd developed anxiety and become prone to chronic infections. She said she felt so tired and anxious that she couldn't do anything beyond getting to work, picking up her kids after school, and stopping somewhere for take-out food before going home. She was tired all day and wanted to lie down and rest by noon. To get through her day, she started drinking more coffee and eating lots of high-carb, sugary foods for energy. In the evening, she usually drank a couple of glasses of wine to relax, and by 7 p.m. her fatigue was so overwhelming that she had to lie down. Needless to say, she didn't get any exercise.

She felt isolated, too. After her divorce, she felt guilty whenever she left her kids with a sitter, so she rarely went out with friends. After years of Lauren turning down her friends' invitations to dinner, movies, or other get-togethers, they'd mostly given up on her.

What finally got her to the clinic was a case of pneumonia that had lingered for several months. She returned to work too soon and had a relapse, and she started to worry about being able to take care of her children.

Lauren's lab tests showed adrenal fatigue. Her cortisol levels were suppressed and her cortisol profile was almost flat, with a much lower morning peak than normal and very low cortisol in the afternoon and evening. This was consistent with Lauren's report of a noticeable drop in energy in the afternoon and severe fatigue in the evening. She was started on 25 milligrams (mg) of supplemental bioidentical cortisol (hydrocortisone) per day for three months to rebuild her adrenals, taking 10 mg first thing in the morning and 5 mg every four hours thereafter.

We recommended that she change her diet to include protein, complex carbohydrates, and healthy fats at every meal and to limit her intake of caffeine, alcohol, and refined carbohydrates. She agreed to start exercising, but because of her debilitated condition and her work schedule, she could only start with a slow, fifteen-minute walk three times a week. She planned to do more as she started feeling stronger. She also agreed to set aside several hours a week just for herself. She hired a babysitter and signed up for a divorce support group, where she met some great women whom she started going out with regularly.

After three months, Lauren's energy level was much improved. The supplemental cortisol, along with her new diet and exercise program, had a noticeable effect. She no longer craved caffeine, alcohol, and refined carbohydrates. She cut out caffeine entirely and cut back to only one or two glasses of wine on weekends.

Once she was feeling better, she was asked to stop taking her supplemental cortisol for four days to see if her adrenal function had improved, as it's common to regain full function within a few months. However, she became very fatigued again, and her three-month follow-up lab tests showed that she still had significantly low cortisol levels. She continued taking supplemental cortisol for another six months. By the ninth month, Lauren was up to forty-five minutes of walking five days per week. She'd continued to significantly improve her diet, being sure to eat meat or fish at least once a day, along with lots of complex carbs and good fats. Her energy levels returned to what she'd experienced in her early thirties, and her anxiety was completely gone. She looked healthy and rested and now had a full life, rounded out by supportive friends and weekly yoga and meditation classes.

IT'S NEVER TOO LATE

Like Lauren, many of us experience multiple symptoms of adrenal fatigue without having the faintest clue that they're caused by adrenal dysfunction. When you're busy with your daily life, it's easy to write your symptoms off. You might find yourself making statement like these: "I'm just tired because I'm almost forty." "I've been working too much." "The commute is draining." "The kids' activities are overwhelming." "I'm not sleeping well." And the list goes on.

But it isn't normal to be tired much of the time, have chronic aches and pains, gain weight, feel weak, lose muscle and sex drive, and not be able to sleep well. You may start looking for individual solutions for each problem: sleeping pills if you're not sleeping well, painkillers if you have aching muscles and joints, antidepressants if your mood is low, weight-loss drugs if you gain weight, you get the idea. It's generally a good idea to stop trying to medicate every symptom individually and instead find the root cause of your symptoms, which will allow you to resolve them for good.

No matter what the cause of adrenal fatigue, it's virtually never too late to resurrect your adrenal function. I know. All of my adrenal hormone levels were incredibly low by the time I was diagnosed with multiple sclerosis. Yet I healed my adrenals and turned my health around. Most would have said that it was too late for me, that MS isn't reversible. But not only do I feel great, my most recent MRI showed no remaining lesions in my brain—one of the hallmark symptoms of MS. Taking bioidentical cortisol (hydrocortisone) to rebuild my adrenal function played a big part in my recovery.

This approach offers great promise for many other diseases that fall into the "too late" category: lupus, fibromyalgia, rheumatoid arthritis, and more. All of these have been shown to have an adrenal component and can potentially be remediated or possibly even resolved by detecting and treating adrenal hormone deficiencies, along with any other related endocrine imbalances, such as hypothyroidism.

WHERE DOES THIS LEAVE US?

You now know what deficient production of adrenal hormones can do to your body, and your symptom evaluation should have given you a good idea as to whether your adrenals are fatigued. If your score on the symptom evaluation is cause for concern, it's time to take the next steps: Do the easy home tests outlined in the next chapter and get the appropriate lab tests (also described in chapter 4), to help determine whether you have adrenal fatigue.

Taking control of your health requires knowledge, discipline, and an understanding of your body's individual needs. Evaluating your adrenal health and finding out whether your adrenals are producing too much or too little cortisol and other adrenal hormones is an effort that will reward you a million times over. This is the next important step in optimizing your adrenal health.

KEY POINTS

- Adrenal fatigue can be caused or exacerbated by too much physical or emotional stress for too long, hypothyroidism, autoimmune activity of adrenal antibodies, a problem with your pituitary or hypothalamus, infections, congenital or hereditary factors, vitamin D deficiency, and synthetic cortisol-like drugs.

- Adrenal fatigue generally develops slowly. In the early stages, the adrenals produce enough cortisol for everyday activities but not enough to handle stressful situations. As the condition progresses, the adrenals can't even make enough for day-to-day activities.

- Looking at symptoms gives valuable insight into the status of your adrenal function; however, remember that many of the symptoms of deficient levels of adrenal hormones are similar to symptoms of excessive levels.

- Insufficient levels of adrenal hormones can cause problems with energy level, weight, aging, immune function, neurotransmitter function, sleep, behavior, cognitive ability, blood pressure, and balance of water, sodium, and potassium.

- Adrenal fatigue can be reversed and adrenal function rebuilt even if adrenal fatigue is severe or long-standing. Conditions like lupus, fibromyalgia, rheumatoid arthritis, and multiple sclerosis all have an adrenal component, and treating underlying adrenal insufficiency may ameliorate symptoms.

CHAPTER 4

Testing Adrenal Function

If your symptom evaluations indicate that you may have adrenal dysfunction, it's time to do a few simple tests at home and then work with your doctor to get lab tests to measure levels of key adrenal hormones. The lab tests and easy home tests outlined in this chapter will give you and your doctor valuable information as to how high or how low your levels of these hormones are. This information is necessary for treating and resolving your symptoms.

Finding the right doctor to help you through this process is critical. Don't underestimate the importance of choosing a doctor with in-depth knowledge and experience in evaluating adrenal function. Doctors who are well versed in this field understand the importance of adrenal evaluation and testing; they know that cortisol needs to be measured in a specific way and that it's also important to measure levels of aldosterone, DHEA, pregnenolone, ACTH, and thyroid hormones, and possibly conduct other tests.

The symptoms in chapters 2 and 3 point to excessive or deficient levels of adrenal hormones. However, factors like vitamin and mineral deficiencies or low levels of sex hormones, such as estrogen or testosterone, can also cause some of these symptoms. To pinpoint the problem you need to have lab tests, but first try the following easy tests you can do at home, as they can help confirm whether adrenal dysfunction is an issue for you.

SELF-TESTS YOU CAN DO AT HOME

The three simple home tests that follow can help you determine whether you have adrenal fatigue. If they're positive for low adrenal function, it will strengthen your case in requesting further investigation by your doctor. Then, once lab tests have determined your specific levels of the different adrenal hormones as well as other related hormones, like sex hormones and thyroid hormones, your doctor can help you determine the right treatment.

Blood Pressure Test

When you have low adrenal function, you generally have low blood pressure, or hypotension. Also common in adrenal fatigue is *postural hypotension*, where your blood pressure drops instead of increases when you rise from lying or sitting down to standing up. The blood pressure test is recognized by adrenal health specialists as indicative of low adrenal function. Postural hypotension is easy to detect; all you need is a blood pressure monitor.

Lie down and relax for at least five minutes, then take your blood pressure while still lying flat. Next, stand up and take your blood pressure again right away. When you stand, your blood pressure should go up. If your diastolic blood pressure (the bottom reading) instead drops more than 10 mm, you may have adrenal fatigue.

This increase in blood pressure while lying down may be one reason why many people with adrenal fatigue find it hard to fall asleep. Until you've treated your adrenal fatigue and reversed your postural hypotension, try propping pillows behind you so you're semireclining for at least fifteen minutes when you go to bed. Fall asleep in this position if possible.

Pupil Contraction Test

One sign of adrenal fatigue, detected in the early 1900s before sophisticated lab tests were available, is when the pupils of the eyes don't hold a steady contraction when exposed to light. This explains why many people with adrenal fatigue are bothered by bright sunlight.

To detect this condition, shine a flashlight past your eye in a dark room while looking in a mirror. Your pupil should contract and remain contracted. If it contracts for a moment, then partially dilates and contracts, or simply gives up and remains dilated, it's indicative of adrenal fatigue.

White Line Test

In the early 1900s, French doctor Émile Sergent found that adrenal fatigue could cause the skin on the abdomen to change color when scratched. All you need for this test is a ballpoint pen.

Using the dull end of the pen, make a mark about six inches long across your abdomen (don't press overly hard or scratch the skin). If your adrenals are functioning normally, the mark will turn from white to red within about ten seconds. If your adrenals are fatigued, however, the line will widen and stay white for about two minutes.

This test isn't a terribly accurate indicator, as only about 40 percent of people with low adrenal function test positive. It generally tests positive only if the adrenal fatigue is fairly severe. So if you do test positive, it's almost certain that you have low adrenal function (J. Wilson 2001).

LAB TESTS FOR ADRENAL FUNCTION

To get a complete understanding of your adrenal status, you should have your levels of cortisol, aldosterone, DHEA, pregnenolone, and ACTH tested. Because many adrenal hormones are made from progesterone, the higher progesterone levels that occur in the second half of the menstrual cycle can raise levels of adrenal hormones in women. It's important to gauge your lowest hormone levels, so women who are still menstruating should have adrenal tests on days 1 through 12 of their cycle (day 1 being the first day of the menstrual period) to determine the lowest levels of adrenal hormones. Men and postmenopausal women can do the tests anytime. On the day of testing, avoid all caffeine, chocolate, sugar, and salt.

Levels of sodium, potassium, calcium, and glucose should also be tested. If you have low levels of sodium and glucose and high levels of potassium and calcium, adrenal fatigue is likely.

Testing Cortisol Levels

Cortisol levels can be tested in blood, urine, saliva, and, infrequently, hair. It's important to test your level several times over the course of a day to determine your production pattern.

There is one important caveat when testing cortisol levels. If you have hypothyroidism (see chapter 6 for more details), cortisol tests may not accurately reflect your adrenal status. Hypothyroidism causes the body to reduce production of cortisol. At the same time, it slows liver function, which decreases the rate at which cortisol is cleared from the body. This results in blood levels of cortisol remaining within the normal range even though the adrenals are fatigued, since the decrease in production is offset by the decrease in clearance from the body (Gordon and Southren 1977).

If you have hypothyroidism, you should have your cortisol levels measured a month or two after you start taking thyroid hormone replacement medication. Once your metabolic rate increases, your body will start to clear cortisol more effectively, allowing low cortisol production and adrenal fatigue to be detected.

BLOOD TESTING

The most widely used test for cortisol is a total cortisol blood test. The drawback to using this method is that it indicates only your total level of cortisol, not the *free level*—the amount that's available for use by your cells, or *bioavailable*. So with blood tests, always make sure that your free cortisol level is measured.

Also, cortisol levels change dramatically during the day, so it's extremely important to test your production pattern as well. If your doctor prefers to do blood tests, make sure to do at least two blood tests on the same day. Do the first one about an hour after you wake up (or when the lab opens), after fasting overnight, and do the second in the midafternoon, about 3 to 4 p.m. This establishes whether your level is high enough in the morning and lower but not too low in the afternoon. Unfortunately, this is inconvenient; it also doesn't give you important nighttime levels, so consider doing a saliva test if possible.

Optimal Blood *Free* Cortisol Levels (Hertoghe 2006)

𝄞   Morning: 20 ng/ml

𝄞   Afternoon: 10 to 12 ng/ml

SALIVA TESTING

Saliva testing for cortisol provides the most useful information. Not only does it show the rhythm of your cortisol production, it also measures free cortisol. It's common for people to have normal levels of total cortisol on blood tests but show low levels on saliva tests because of this bioavailability issue.

Saliva testing can be done anywhere. You simply collect saliva in cotton and seal it in a tube. Most testing labs recommend measuring levels four to six times during the day, including 8 a.m., noon, 4 p.m., 8 p.m., midnight, and 4 a.m. The night samples are particularly important, as adrenal fatigue often causes a disrupted circadian rhythm of cortisol production that results in elevated cortisol at night.

Dr. Michael Borkin, the research director at Sabre Sciences, a company that offers saliva testing, has conducted extensive research into what changing levels of cortisol throughout the day tell us about our adrenal function, and how the elevations or decreases in cortisol levels at different points during the day can show where stress is originating. In a personal communication, he explained that the cortisol level at 8 a.m. gives insight into the size and status of your adrenal glands. If your adrenals are enlarged, indicting that they're in overdrive, you'll have high cortisol levels. If your adrenals are atrophied or shrinking, you're on your way to adrenal fatigue and your levels will be low.

Dr. Borkin also said that the drop from 8 a.m. to noon can indicate an inflammatory process. A drop of 50 percent or more is usually associated with problems with the digestive system, while a drop in excess of 70 percent usually indicates a parasitic infestation. The noon measurement is especially reflective of blood sugar control, and levels at 4 p.m. give insight into chronic infections, with elevated levels generally indicating bacterial overgrowth, and low levels indicating viral infections. Cortisol levels at 8 p.m. are associated with the ability to utilize insulin and can indicate insulin resistance or type 2 diabetes. The midnight measurement is important because elevated cortisol at this time can interfere with the release of growth hormone and proper immune function. Spiking at 4 a.m., which is abnormal, shows that blood sugar reserves have run out, so the adrenals have increased their output of cortisol to bring blood sugar levels back into normal range.

Optimal Saliva Cortisol Levels (Hertoghe 2006)

- Morning: 20 to 30 nmol/l (nanomoles per liter)

- Noon: 7 to 11 nmol/l

- Evening: 6 to 9 nmol/l

- Night: 5 nmol/l

URINE TESTING

A twenty-four-hour urine test for cortisol gives your total amount of free cortisol output over a twenty-four-hour period. However, it won't detect a disrupted production pattern. It involves collecting all of your urine during a twenty-four-hour period, so you need to do it when you can stay near the collection container (which must be kept refrigerated) most of the day.

Optimal Twenty-Four-Hour Urine Cortisol Levels (Hertoghe 2006)

- 70 mcg (micrograms)

Testing Aldosterone Levels

Aldosterone testing is done with a blood test or twenty-four-hour urine test. To get a complete picture of your aldosterone status, your doctor may also test your levels of sodium, potassium, and renin. *Renin* is a kidney enzyme that stimulates production of aldosterone. Renin levels go up when aldosterone levels decline.

Levels of both aldosterone and renin become elevated when the body is struggling to conserve sodium and fluid. High aldosterone levels cause the kidneys to reabsorb more sodium and release more potassium, which can cause an electrolyte imbalance. Low aldosterone levels, which can occur when adrenal function is deficient, cause dehydration, low blood pressure, and low blood levels of sodium and potassium.

Both aldosterone and renin levels are highest in the morning, so testing should be done first thing, while still fasting. Aldosterone levels are affected by a person's position while blood is drawn (this is taken into account when interpreting results), as well as stress and the amount of sodium in the diet, so avoid salt for twenty-four hours before the test. Levels can also be affected by a variety of medications, including diuretics, steroids, oral contraceptives, analgesics like ibuprofen, and heart medications, including beta-blockers and angiotensin-converting enzyme (ACE) inhibitors. Make sure that your doctor is aware of any medications you're taking before testing.

Optimal Aldosterone Blood Levels (Hertoghe 2006)

- Aldosterone: greater than 15 ng/dl (nanograms per deciliter) if blood is drawn while sitting; or greater than approximately 7 if blood is drawn while lying down

- Sodium: 141 nmol/l

- Potassium: 4.3 mmol/l (millimoles per liter)

- Renin: a ratio of aldosterone to renin greater than 25 is suggestive of hyper-aldosteronism

Testing DHEA Levels

DHEA levels can also get too high or two low. The form of DHEA usually measured by tests is DHEA-sulfate, which can be measured in either blood or saliva. Low levels of DHEA-sulfate indicate low adrenal function. DHEA blood tests are done first thing in the morning, while still fasting. Saliva testing is done using the same samples taken for testing cortisol levels.

Optimal Levels of DHEA (Hertoghe 2006)

- Women: In blood, 280 mcg/dl (micrograms per deciliter); in saliva, 200 pg/ml

- Men: In blood, 400 mcg/dl; in saliva, 250 pg/ml

Testing Pregnenolone Levels

Levels of pregnenolone, an important adrenal hormone as well as a precursor to many other hormones, should be measured for a complete picture of adrenal health. Pregnenolone helps normalize cortisol levels, bringing them down if they're high and raising them if they're low. It can be converted into many different hormones, particularly cortisol and DHEA. If your levels are low and you decide to take supplemental pregnenolone, measure levels of all three hormones—pregnenolone, cortisol, and DHEA—after a month or two of supplementation to ensure they're not getting too high or out of balance.

Optimal Blood Level of Pregnenolone

- 50 to 200 ng/dl

Testing ACTH Levels

ACTH is a pituitary hormone that stimulates your adrenals to produce cortisol, DHEA, and aldosterone. ACTH is produced in a pattern somewhat similar to that of cortisol: highest in the morning between 6 and 8 a.m., and lowest in the evening between 6 and 11 p.m. Testing ACTH levels will determine whether low production of these hormones is caused by pituitary dysfunction or a problem with your adrenals themselves. If your ACTH is elevated but your cortisol is low, your adrenals are the problem. Your pituitary is sending the right signals, but your adrenals are too tired to respond.

If both ACTH and cortisol are low, it indicates a problem with your pituitary function. Your pituitary should detect low cortisol levels and increase ACTH to stimulate production. If both ACTH and cortisol are low, be sure to test levels of the other hormones controlled by the pituitary, including testosterone for men, estrogen and progesterone for women, growth hormone, and thyroid hormones (TSH, free T3, and free T4—more on these in chapter 6). If your pituitary has been damaged, which can often occur due to head trauma, these hormones will also generally need to be supplemented.

Your doctor may test cortisol first and, if it's low, test ACTH and also do an ACTH stimulation test to assess your adrenal glands' response to stress. In this test, baseline cortisol levels are tested, then ACTH is injected and cortisol is measured again after thirty and sixty minutes to see how your adrenals are responding. If they're functioning properly, your cortisol level should double within sixty minutes. Although this test can diagnose Addison's disease and pituitary impairment, it often fails to detect adrenal fatigue, so don't rely on it as the final word on your adrenal health.

Optimal Blood Level of ACTH (Hertoghe 2006)

    45 mg/l

CRH Stimulation Test

If your ACTH test result was abnormal, a CRH stimulation test can help determine the cause of your adrenal insufficiency. For this test, blood cortisol level is measured, then synthetic corticotropin-releasing hormone, the hypothalamic hormone that stimulates release of ACTH from the pituitary gland, is injected. Cortisol is then measured 30, 60, 90, and 120 minutes after the injection.

People with Addison's disease produce elevated levels of ACTH but no cortisol because the adrenals are too tired to respond. In people with secondary adrenal insufficiency, the ACTH response is absent or delayed because CRH can't stimulate ACTH secretion if your pituitary is damaged.

This test, or an ACTH stimulation test, is also used to diagnose mild congenital adrenal hyperplasia. After CRH stimulation, people suffering from mild adrenal hyperplasia with a deficiency of 21-hydroxylase enzyme, the most common enzyme deficiency in this condition, have significantly lower levels of free cortisol and higher levels of ACTH and 17-hydroxyprogesterone, a cortisol precursor.

Testing for Adrenal Antibodies

Adrenal antibodies, also called adrenocortical antibodies, are directed against the adrenal cortex—the outer layer of the adrenal glands. These antibodies destroy adrenal tissue, interfere with hormone production, and can ultimately lead to Addison's disease. You should have an antibody blood test if you have a family history of Addison's disease or extreme symptoms of adrenal fatigue.

Leslie's Story

At age thirty-eight, Leslie was a case study in adrenal fatigue when she came to the clinic. She had symptoms of long-standing cortisol deficiency, including chronic fatigue, brain fog, worsening allergies, sleep problems, psoriasis, chronic constipation, and a very thin face, giving her a gaunt, tired look. She was exhausted throughout the day, having a hard time getting up in the morning and then struggling to get through work.

As a bookkeeper, Leslie did a lot of detail work. She was worried she would have to quit her job because she was starting to make a lot of mistakes. She was having a hard time concentrating, and her memory was getting bad.

In her health history Leslie disclosed that she had suffered a serious concussion when she fell off a horse as a teenager. Head injuries are a significant risk factor for pituitary dysfunction, so we tested her adrenal function as well as levels of sex hormones, growth hormone, and thyroid hormones.

While waiting for the lab results to come back, she did the home adrenal tests as well as a basal body temperature test to assess her metabolic rate and thyroid function (described in chapter 6) and reported that they indicated low adrenal and thyroid function. She had consistently low basal body temperature (see chapter 6) for ten days. She also had postural hypotension and was positive for adrenal fatigue on the white line and pupil contraction tests.

Leslie's lab tests confirmed that she had adrenal and thyroid deficiencies. Her cortisol levels were suppressed at all four points during the day. She also had low ACTH, indicating that her pituitary wasn't functioning correctly. Her DHEA, pregnenolone, and aldosterone levels were also low, as were levels of other hormones controlled by the pituitary, including thyroid, growth hormone, estradiol, progesterone, and insulin.

Leslie clearly had pituitary damage, probably from her head injury. Her low hormone levels required an initial replacement protocol consisting of a 0.1 mg estradiol patch all month, with 100 mg of progesterone in the last two weeks of her cycle, thyroid hormone therapy, 5 mg of hydrocortisone every four hours, 0.2 mg of growth hormone by subcutaneous injection every morning, and 5 mg of oral DHEA every morning.

A month later, a more energetic and smiling Leslie reported that although it was still hard to get going in the morning, she was able to get through her workday with a clear mind and good concentration. She was sleeping better and excited that her psoriasis was shrinking and was less itchy and sore. Her constipation had also resolved completely, but she was concerned because her symptoms had started to return after a week.

However, this made sense. Because her body had adapted to its new, higher metabolic level, she needed a higher dose of thyroid hormones, as well as more cortisol for a robust early morning cortisol peak. Her dosage of thyroid medication was increased and her early morning cortisol dosage was raised to 10 mg.

When Leslie came in for her six-month appointment, her symptoms were almost completely resolved. Her allergies were finally subsiding, her psoriasis was barely detectable, she had plenty of energy, and she was sleeping well, without waking in the night. Now that she was stabilized, she was excited about meeting with the nutritionist to design a diet and exercise plan, and continuing on the path to rebuilding her health.

Testing for Hormone Imbalances That Can Contribute to Adrenal Dysfunction

The following additional tests are valuable in detecting hormone imbalances and deficiencies that can negatively affect your adrenal function.

WOMEN'S SEX HORMONES

Remember, the body sees deficient levels of sex hormones as a stressor and responds by pumping out cortisol, so it's also important to test levels of sex hormones to get a complete picture of your hormone status. Testing for women should include levels of estradiol (estrogen), progesterone, and testosterone.

Postmenopausal women can be tested any day; those who are still ovulating should be tested on day 21 of their menstrual cycle. This is the secondary peak level of estradiol (after the peak at ovulation) and the peak level of progesterone. Testing at this time will also tell you if you ovulated that month. In cycles where you don't ovulate, you don't make progesterone, so its level remains low.

It's also important to measure levels of sex-hormone-binding globulin (SHBG). When levels are high, it binds a lot of the body's sex hormones, leading to symptoms of hormone deficiency even if your body is actually producing sufficient amounts.

Optimal Blood Levels of Sex Hormones for Women (Hertoghe 2006)

- Estradiol: greater than 120 pg/ml

- Progesterone (luteal phase, or second half of menstrual cycle): 13 to 23 ng/ml

- Progesterone (follicular phase, or first half of menstrual cycle): 1.4 ng/ml

🦶 SHBG: 65 nmol/l

🦶 Testosterone: 35 ng/dl

MEN'S SEX HORMONES

Just as with female sex hormones, loss of sex hormones in men also triggers cortisol release, so their levels should be measured to give a complete picture of hormone health. Testing for men should include levels of testosterone (free and total levels), progesterone, and the two primary hormones made from testosterone—dihydrotestosterone (DHT) and estradiol (estrogen). The ratio between DHT and estradiol gives a more complete picture of hormone function and health. DHT is more active than testosterone, and high levels can cause prostate enlargement. But low levels in relationship to estradiol are also bad, as DHT protects against the inflammatory effects of estradiol, blocking estradiol's proliferative effects on tissues.

Studies show that prostate problems, the bane of so many aging men, can be caused by either too much DHT or too much estradiol (Keith, Nicholson, and Assinder 2006). That's where progesterone comes in; it can balance both DHT and estradiol. If your level of progesterone is low and levels of DHT or estradiol are high, supplementing with progesterone can balance excess DHT and estradiol.

If testosterone levels are low, luteinizing hormone (LH) and follicle-stimulating hormone (FSH) should also be tested. Levels of these two hormones, made by the pituitary, will indicate whether low testosterone is caused by a problem with the pituitary or with the testes. If these two levels are low, it indicates a problem with the pituitary, which should be making more LH and FSH to stimulate testosterone production. If their levels are high and testosterone is low, then the problem is with the testes, which aren't responding properly to the message being sent by the pituitary.

Optimal Blood Levels of Sex Hormones for Men (Hertoghe 2006)

🦶 Total testosterone: 700 ng/dl

🦶 Free testosterone: 250 pg/ml

🦶 DHT: 70 ng/dl

🦶 Estradiol: 25 pg/ml

🦶 Progesterone: 1.2 ng/ml

🦶 LH: 3 mIU/ml (milli–international units per milliliter); over 8 is too high

🦶 FSH: 2 mIU/ml; over 7 is too high

THYROID HORMONES

Because of the close reciprocal relationship between adrenal and thyroid function, it's important to test thyroid hormone levels if you suspect adrenal dysfunction. Thyroid function testing for both men and women should include tests for levels of TSH, free T3, free T4, and reverse T3. Chapter 6 will provide details on thyroid testing.

Optimal Thyroid Hormone Levels (Hertoghe 2006)

- TSH: 1 mIU/ml

- Free T3: 2.5 to 3.4 pg/ml

- Free T4: 1.3 to 1.8 ng/dl

- Reverse T3: less than 25 ng/dl

INSULIN, GLUCOSE, AND HEMOGLOBIN A1C

Fasting insulin and glucose levels should be measured as part of a complete adrenal evaluation, since levels are affected by adrenal dysfunction and imbalanced cortisol levels. Hemoglobin A1c (HbA1c) is also very helpful, offering a picture of your average blood glucose level for the past few months. If you have elevated fasting insulin levels, it's likely that you are, or are on your way to becoming, insulin resistant.

Optimal Levels of Insulin, Glucose, and HBA1c (Hertoghe 2006)

- Fasting insulin: 4 to 9 micro-IU/ml

- Fasting glucose: 80 to 95 mg/dl

- HbA1c: 4.5 to 6.0%

GROWTH HORMONE

If ACTH tests show deficient pituitary function, have your levels of growth hormone tested. Because the body makes growth hormone primarily in the middle of the night, it's not practical to measure it directly. However, you can obtain an accurate assessment of growth hormone status by measuring levels of insulin-like growth factor (IGF-1), a hormone produced when the liver is stimulated by human growth hormone. It's also important to measure its binding protein, IGFBP3, which is also an important hormone in its own right.

Optimal Levels for Growth Hormone Tests (Hertoghe 2006)

- IGF-1: 300 ng/ml

- IGFBP3: 3 mg/l

VITAMIN D

There are two types of vitamin D: vitamin D_2, found in foods from plant sources, and vitamin D_3, or cholecalciferol, found in animal products. Vitamin D_3 has more biologic activity, so that's the form that's tested and best for supplementation. Its precursor 25-hydroxyvitamin D_3 is a better marker of vitamin D reserves than the more active form, 1,25-dihydroxyvitamin D_3, and more predictive of good health. Also, blood levels of 1,25-dihydroxyvitamin D_3 are often normal even when the precursor is deficient (Armas, Hollis, and Heaney 2004).

Levels of vitamin D fluctuate with the season, rising abruptly in June and remaining high until October (Brot et al. 2001). The fluctuation may be related to the number of hours of sunshine per month, with a two-month time lag. Ideally, you should have your vitamin D levels tested sometime between September and March, when levels are at their lowest.

Optimal level of 25-hydroxyvitamin D_3 (Gorham et al. 2007)

ⵏ Over 55 ng/ml

WHERE DOES THIS LEAVE US?

You've done a great job getting here. It's been a lot of work analyzing your symptoms and having lab tests, but you're almost done. You've found a doctor experienced in adrenal function, the final results are in, and at last you know whether your adrenals are making too few or too many hormones.

This explains so much. It isn't all in your head. Your adrenal glands are at the root of all those mysterious complaints you've been telling doctor after doctor about for years. The rest is easy. It doesn't matter whether your levels of adrenal hormones are too low or too high; both conditions respond well to the approaches outlined in the rest of the book. In chapter 5, you'll learn how to reduce or bolster your hormone levels naturally, using nutritional approaches or supplemental bio-identical hormones. Once you and your doctor have figured out the right treatment plan, you'll be feeling better sooner than you think!

KEY POINTS

❧ Finding a doctor experienced in the field of testing and treating adrenal problems is critical; these doctors understand which tests are necessary to detect adrenal problems and are familiar with the treatments that can optimize your adrenal function.

❧ There are several tests you can do at home to identify adrenal fatigue: the blood pressure test, the pupil contraction test, and the white line test. Try them at home and tell your doctor about the results.

❧ Have lab tests for levels of adrenal hormones, including cortisol (preferably in saliva, measured four to six times over the course of a day), aldosterone, DHEA-sulfate, pregnenolone, and ACTH, as well as a corticotropin-releasing hormone stimulation test if necessary.

❧ Additional recommended tests include adrenal antibodies; women's sex hormones, including estradiol, progesterone, SHBG, and testosterone; men's sex hormones, including free and total testosterone, DHT, and estradiol; thyroid hormones, including TSH and free T3 and T4; insulin, glucose, and hemoglobin A1c; growth hormone; and vitamin D.

CHAPTER 5

Restoring Adrenal Health Naturally

By now you've completed all the adrenal health symptom questionnaires and home testing. Even if you haven't yet found a doctor to test your hormone levels, you probably have a good idea how your adrenals are functioning. If you've detected signs and symptoms of adrenal dysfunction, the next step is to chart a path back to optimal adrenal health. Even if you lack the financial resources to work with a specialist or have severe or long-standing adrenal dysfunction, there's a lot you can do right away to support and rebuild your adrenals.

In this chapter, we'll take a look at ways to curb excess cortisol production and then look at ways to rebuild fatigued adrenals. But first, you should know that certain vitamins and minerals are vital to optimal adrenal function and will help no matter what your adrenal issue is. You can take these nutrients as supplements, or get them from food:

- **B vitamins:** Food sources include whole grains and some beans, peas, and nuts. Nutritional yeast is another good source, and the only good vegetarian source of B_{12}, which is naturally found only in meat, fish, and dairy products.

- **Vitamin C:** Food sources include most fruits and vegetables, especially citrus, papaya, cantaloupe, strawberries, bell peppers, broccoli, tomatoes, and dark leafy greens.

- **Magnesium:** Food sources include dark leafy greens, whole grains, and most nuts, seeds, and legumes.

- **Zinc:** Food sources include most meats, seafood, and poultry, and, to a lesser extent, whole grains, nuts, and seeds.

REDUCING EXCESS CORTISOL PRODUCTION

If your cortisol is elevated, it's important to reduce it to within normal range. In chapter 2, you saw the damage that can be caused by elevated cortisol, including high blood pressure and elevated cholesterol, triglycerides, insulin, and blood sugar. The primary way to reduce levels of all your adrenal hormones, whether cortisol, adrenaline, DHEA, or aldosterone, is through exercise, diet, and lifestyle modification, including stress management. However, certain herbs, vitamins, minerals, and other supplements can also help reduce levels of these hormones and restore balance to your adrenal function, as can acupuncture and massage.

Just be aware that some products touted as natural solutions may not have been proven effective. For example, supplements containing magnolia bark extract are sold as cortisol-lowering products for weight loss (brand names include CortiSlim, Relacore, and Relora). Although these supplements have been proven safe, a 2008 study of Relora showed no change in participant cortisol levels after taking 750 mg daily for six weeks (Kalman et al. 2008). On the other had, all of the following have been proven effective in lowering cortisol levels.

Acupuncture and Massage

Studies show that acupuncture can reduce excess cortisol production. A Chinese study looked at a group of people undergoing surgery. Combined with general anesthesia, acupuncture helped control cortisol levels so they didn't get too high and cause tissue damage, or too low, which would trigger chronic inflammation (Yang, Hang, and Sun 2001). Acupuncture can also decrease high levels of aldosterone and renin, helping to lower high blood pressure (Li, Shen, and Peng 2005). These results suggest that acupuncture has regulatory effects on electrolyte balance as well as stress hormone levels. In addition, many studies have shown that massage helps reduce cortisol levels (Field et al. 2005).

Vitamins, Minerals, and Other Supplements

The following vitamins, minerals, and other supplements have been proven to reduce cortisol levels. Note that the nutrients you get from food are best; most foods contain combinations of nutrients that work together synergistically. For that reason, try to get the nutrients you need from foods whenever possible. Ideally, you should work with a nutritionist or health practitioner to measure your levels of key vitamins and minerals and detect deficiencies. This will allow you to develop an optimal individualized treatment program.

Chromium. Chromium helps the body metabolize carbohydrates for energy and works with insulin to allow glucose to enter your cells. Chromium deficiency causes glucose to build up in the blood. Because chromium plays a role in balancing blood sugar, it can also help control the spike of cortisol that occurs if glucose levels fall too low at night. Brewer's yeast is a good source of chromium. The generally recommended dose is 250 to 500 mg twice per day.

Fish oil. Fish oil has been shown to lower cortisol levels. In one study, participants who took 7.2 grams of fish oil per day for three weeks had lower cortisol levels, heart rate, and blood pressure (Delarue et al. 2003). The best food sources are oily fish like sardines, salmon, trout, mackerel, and anchovies, which store fat in their bodies. Because cod store fat in the liver, cod liver oil is potentially a good source. But since they also store fat-soluble vitamins A and D in their livers, cod liver oil contains high concentrations of these vitamins, which can be toxic in high quantities, so be careful not to overdo cod liver oil supplements. If you take a fish oil supplement, those made from the whole bodies of fish are a better choice. Unfortunately, oily fish generally contain higher levels of contaminants too, so try to buy fish from less polluted waters, such as off the coast of Alaska or New Zealand. The generally recommended dose is 1,000 to 4,000 mg per day.

Magnesium. Studies show that magnesium supplementation decreases serum cortisol levels after aerobic exercise (Golf et al. 1984). The generally recommended dose is 1,000 mg per day or to bowel tolerance.

Melatonin. Melatonin, a hormone made in the pineal gland, regulates your circadian rhythm, or biological clock, as well as sleep. Melatonin is much lower in people with elevated cortisol. Studies have shown that melatonin supplementation modulates cortisol production (Zisapel, Tarrasch, and Laudon 2005). As with all other hormones, it's best to use the lowest effective dose. Start at 0.5 mg fifteen minutes before bed, and raise the dosage, if need be, until you are sleeping more soundly. Always take melatonin sublingually (under your tongue), as opposed to swallowing it. As with all hormones, it's best to work with a health practitioner when taking supplemental melatonin.

Phosphatidylserine. In a study of healthy men, 800 mg of phosphatidylserine per day significantly reduced cortisol during physical stress (Monteleone et al. 1992). In another study, participants who took 400 to 600 mg of phosphatidylserine daily and participated in stressful activities (math tests, job interviews, and the like) had a significant reduction of the cortisol response (Hellhammer et al. 2004). In the body's tissues, phosphatidylserine converts into phosphorylated serine, so supplementing with phosphorylated serine is another effective way to temper cortisol. Phosphatidylserine is difficult to get from food, as the primary sources are cow brains and soy lecithin (which must be consumed in impractically high doses). The generally recommended dose is 300 to 800 mg per day.

Vitamin C. Vitamin C has been shown to help reduce elevated cortisol. In a study involving long-distance runners, athletes who took 1,500 mg of vitamin C per day had significantly lower cortisol levels after running a marathon than those who took much lower doses or a placebo (Peters et al. 2001). In another study, participants who took 3,000 mg per day experienced a decrease in cortisol levels and blood pressure, as well as their perception of stress (Brody et al. 2002). Vitamin C is found in many fruits and vegetables: bell peppers, broccoli, oranges, strawberries, cabbage, brussels sprouts, dark leafy greens, and tomatoes. Start with a dose of 1,000 mg per day and increase to bowel tolerance or as much as 3,000 mg per day.

Herbs

Several herbs have been proven to reduce cortisol levels and the negative effects of stress: ashwagandha, *Ginkgo biloba*, ginseng, maca, and *Rhodiola rosea*.

Ashwagandha. Ashwagandha (*Withania somnifera*) is widely used by Ayurvedic physicians in India. Studies show it lowers cortisol levels during stress (Singh et al. 1982). The generally recommended dose is 250 mg per day.

Ginkgo biloba. Ginkgo has been used for over five thousand years to treat a variety of health conditions, including elevated cortisol levels. In one study, participants under stress who took 120 mg of ginkgo biloba extract per day had smaller increases in their cortisol levels and blood pressure than those who took a placebo (Jezova et al. 2002). The generally recommended dose is 100 to 200 mg per day.

Ginseng. Some herbs are known as adaptogenic because they have the remarkable capacity to restore balance, helping compensate for either overactivity or underactivity of various physiological systems. In the case of the adrenals, ginseng is adaptogenic, either reducing high cortisol or its negative effects or helping raise low cortisol levels, depending on your body's needs. There are several different types of ginseng, and all have been shown to provide protection against both physical and psychological stress (Nocerino, Amato, and Izzo 2000). The generally recommended dose is 100 to 300 mg per day.

Maca root. In animal studies, the turniplike root of the maca plant significantly reduced levels of both cortisol and ACTH. It also appears to stimulate sex hormone production (Meissner et al. 2006). Maca root generally comes as a powder. Talk to your doctor or nutritionist about how much you should take.

Rhodiola rosea. Rhodiola can help control excess cortisol release. Studies have demonstrated its effectiveness in combating both physical and psychological stress (Kelly 2001). The generally recommended dose is 100 to 200 mg per day.

◖ Jan's Story

Jan, age forty-three, came into the clinic because she was concerned she was going into menopause early. She'd started having hot flashes, vaginal dryness, dry skin and hair, and sleeping problems, and she was tired and depressed a lot of the time. Her stomach had also gotten huge in the last year in spite of constant dieting. She'd done daily crunches and started running, but nothing was working.

While researching her symptoms, she'd stumbled onto syndrome X. Reading that it caused obesity around the waist, high cholesterol, high triglycerides, and high blood pressure really scared her. Her cholesterol and triglycerides had been elevated since her late thirties. She had also had high blood pressure at her last physical, so she thought she might have syndrome X.

After looking at her symptom questionnaires and family and personal health histories, we agreed with her. She had all the symptoms of syndrome X, along with a family history of heart disease and type 2 diabetes. In addition, her diet consisted mainly of refined carbohydrates, which kept her insulin and glucose levels constantly elevated.

Jan's tests confirmed that she had syndrome X. Both her fasting and nonfasting insulin and glucose levels were significantly elevated, as was her hemoglobin A1c, indicating that she was insulin resistant and on her way to becoming diabetic. Her cortisol levels were elevated throughout the day and particularly high at night. Her DHEA and aldosterone levels were also elevated.

Jan's estrogen level was fine on day 21 of her menstrual cycle, but her low progesterone level indicated she wasn't ovulating. She asked why she had the symptoms of low estrogen when her levels were okay. We explained that high cortisol had made her brain less sensitive to estrogens, resulting in symptoms of low estrogen. The answer wasn't to supplement estrogen, but to get her cortisol levels under control so her own estrogen would be more available.

Her thyroid was also showing signs of slowing, with elevated levels of thyroid-stimulating hormone and low levels of thyroid hormones, so she started on thyroid hormone therapy. Jan also met with the nutritionist and started a strict diet emphasizing a balanced mix of protein, complex carbs, and healthy fats and eliminating all refined carbs, sugar, and caffeine. She was committed to sticking with the diet, as she had seen her mother struggle with type 2 diabetes for years and didn't want to end up having to use insulin. She continued her exercise routine, but instead of running every day, she cut back to two days a week, did resistance training at the gym two days a week, took a yoga class on the fifth day, and then took two days off.

She also started taking supplements: 2,000 mg of vitamin C, 2,000 mg of fish oil, 1,000 mg of magnesium, 250 mg of ashwagandha, 600 mg of phosphatidylserine, and 0.5 mg of melatonin sublingually at night.

A month later, Jan reported that she was sleeping better and having fewer hot flashes. Her energy was noticeably better and her jeans were looser. By three months, she could fit into pants a full size smaller and her face had lost its puffy look. Her energy returned to normal, and she had very few days when she felt depressed.

By six months all the signs of low estrogen were gone. Her ovulation tester showed she was ovulating every month, and her menstrual cycles had returned to normal. At nine months, Jan's stomach was hardly enlarged at all and she felt like herself again. Her follow-up tests showed normal glucose and HbA1c levels. Her insulin was still a bit elevated but significantly lower than it had been, showing she was well on her way to resolving her insulin resistance. Her cortisol levels were completely normal, with an optimal circadian pattern: high in the morning, getting lower all day long, and staying low at night.

Her cholesterol was still a little high, at 203, but it had come down significantly from 280, and her triglycerides and blood pressure were normal. She had regained her health, and with continued balanced diet, exercise, and thyroid therapy, would probably continue to bring her cholesterol down—and escape her mother's diabetes.

TREATING ADRENAL FATIGUE

Fatigued adrenal glands have the miraculous ability to regain full functionality if given the right support. Diet and lifestyle, discussed in chapters 7 and 8, play a big part in successfully healing the adrenals. In addition, certain vitamins, minerals, herbs, and hormones can be very effective in restoring adrenal function, as can acupuncture.

Supplementing deficient levels of adrenal hormones with their bioidentical equivalent is becoming a widely practiced method of helping restore adrenal function. Low dosages of bioidentical cortisol (hydrocortisone), DHEA, pregnenolone, and aldosterone can give fatigued adrenals a much-needed rest. If your symptoms and test results show deficiencies of any of these key hormones, explore the following treatment options with your doctor.

Acupuncture

Acupuncture can stimulate cortisol production naturally by enhancing adrenal function (Lee et al. 1982). In addition, studies have shown that acupuncture can help with post-traumatic stress disorder (PTSD), which is associated with low cortisol levels (Hollifield et al. 2007).

Vitamins, Minerals, and Other Supplements

Digestive enzymes, pantothenic acid, other B vitamins, phosphatidylserine, sodium, vitamin C, and vitamin D can all support adrenal function and help resolve adrenal fatigue.

DIGESTIVE ENZYMES

Digestive enzymes help break down food in the gastrointestinal tract, making their nutrients accessible. When the adrenals are fatigued, digestion is often impaired, so you may need to take digestive enzymes to get the most benefit from your food.

PANTOTHENIC ACID

Pantothenic acid (vitamin B_5) helps activate the adrenal glands and increase their production of hormones. It also plays a key role in energy metabolism and synthesis of acetylcholine, an important neurotransmitter. Pantothenic acid combats fatigue and strengthens endurance, and studies show that it can assist in resolving adrenal insufficiency (Tarasov, Sheibak, and Moiseenok 1985). Foods rich in pantothenic acid include legumes, whole grains, salmon, cauliflower, broccoli, sweet potatoes, and tomatoes. Many doctors recommend taking 100 mg daily. Because it can disrupt sleep, avoid taking it after 3 p.m.

OTHER B VITAMINS

Other B vitamins are also involved in energy production and necessary for your body to make adrenal hormones. Because the B vitamins work together, it's best to take a B complex supplement. Daily requirements for the different B vitamins vary substantially. Look for B complex supplement with at least 50 mg of vitamins B_1 and B_2 and niacin.

SODIUM

Aldosterone regulates the amount of sodium you retain in your body and how much you excrete. If you have low blood pressure or feel light-headed when you stand up, you may have an electrolyte imbalance caused by low aldosterone levels. Salts rich in minerals, such as sea salt, can help raise blood pressure and counteract low aldosterone. If you have a problem with frequent urination during the night, try using more salt with your evening meal, or drink a glass of water with ½ to 1 teaspoon of salt stirred in at bedtime. Eating more salt doesn't fix the underlying problem of sodium loss caused by low aldosterone levels, but it does temporarily increase the amount of sodium available to your body. If you try to cut back on salt, it can worsen your symptoms of low aldosterone.

VITAMIN C

Vitamin C is essential in the production of adrenal hormones and supporting your immune system. Start with a dose of 1,000 mg per day and increase to bowel tolerance or as much as 3,000 mg per day.

VITAMIN D

Vitamin D deficiency should be corrected by sun exposure, eating foods high in vitamin D, and taking supplemental vitamin D_3. Try to avoid spending much time in semidarkness during the day. Depending on your skin color, you may need more sun exposure to get enough vitamin D. Dark-skinned people need ninety minutes to two hours of light exposure to get the same amount of vitamin D that light-skinned people get in ten to twenty minutes (Matsuoka et al. 1991). Food sources of vitamin D are saturated fats found in foods such as egg yolk, butter, lard, and liver, as well as oily fish. In the United States it's also added to fortified milk, bread, and other wheat products.

Most doctors recommend taking 1,000 to 4,000 IU of vitamin D_3 to start if your levels are low. It's important to measure your levels again after you start taking supplements to see if you're at the right dose. Keep in mind that your need for vitamin D can vary greatly from summer to winter, depending on what latitude you live at and how much sun exposure you get in the winter. Exciting new studies (for example, Burton et al. 2010) are showing the beneficial effect of very high doses of vitamin D (up to 50,000 IU per day) in the treatment of condition such as neuralgia, multiple sclerosis, and musculoskeletal pain.

If you supplement vitamin D, make sure you have enough calcium and magnesium in your diet. Research suggests that you should supplement with 1,000 to 1,200 mg of calcium daily, and supplement magnesium at half the dose of calcium you're taking (Standing Committee on the Scientific Evaluation of Dietary Reference Intakes 1997).

Herbs

Ginseng and licorice can help counteract adrenal fatigue and rebuild adrenal function.

Ginseng. As an adaptogenic herb, ginseng not only reduces the effects of excess cortisol, it can also help restore flagging adrenal function and prevent your adrenals from atrophying. In animal studies it's been found to inhibit adrenal atrophy caused by low cortisol (Tanizawa et al. 1981). Ginseng boosts energy and also helps restore energy reserves by increasing carbohydrate metabolism and glucose storage. In studies of women, ginseng was shown to increase levels of both DHEA and testosterone (Al-Dujaili, Chalmers, and Sharp 2007). Dosing depends on the type of ginseng used, so consult with your doctor or a supplement expert.

Licorice. Licorice helps sustain cortisol levels by slowing its breakdown in the body. For adrenal fatigue, try licorice teas or supplements. Licorice candies contain anise seed and sugar, which taste similar but don't have the same effect on cortisol. However, be aware that licorice root used for too long, or in large doses, can lead to high blood pressure, water retention, and lowered potassium levels. It can even cause breast enlargement in men. So be careful not to overdo it.

Hormone Therapy

If your level of cortisol, DHEA, pregnenolone, progesterone, or aldosterone is deficient, your doctor may recommend that you supplement with bioidentical hormones. This can give your adrenal glands a much-needed rest from the everyday demands of hormone production. Supplementation is the fastest way to raise levels of these key hormones, but it's appropriate only if your levels are significantly deficient or if you've been unsuccessful in raising your levels through diet, nutritional support, and lifestyle modification.

ADRENAL CORTICAL GLANDULAR EXTRACTS

Desiccated adrenal gland extracts have been used to treat adrenal fatigue since the 1800s. They are made from the cortex of bovine adrenal glands and contain very low doses of cortisol, making them helpful in supporting your adrenal glands if you don't have a serious deficiency. Look for a reputable brand like Isocort, made by Bezwecken, to ensure quality, potency, and safety, and consult with your doctor about dosing.

CORTISOL

If your lab tests show significant cortisol deficiency, you may need to supplement cortisol levels temporarily by taking hydrocortisone, which is a synthetic bioidentical form of cortisol. Supplementing with hydrocortisone takes the demand for cortisol production off your adrenal glands and allows them to rest, heal, and regain full function.

Hydrocortisone is short acting and can be given in doses that mimic natural cortisol secretion. The general rule of thumb is to take hydrocortisone for two to three months, and then stop taking it so that you can retest your levels and monitor your symptoms. If your levels have normalized and your symptoms don't reappear, your doctor will generally have you stop taking it. If you haven't regained full adrenal function, you'll probably need to continue taking hydrocortisone, with periodic breaks to monitor your cortisol levels and symptoms until they've resolved. This can take anywhere from a month to several years, depending on how long-standing and severe your deficiency is.

When your adrenal glands are healthy and making optimal levels of cortisol, you produce about 35 to 40 mg of cortisol per day (Jefferies 2004). It's important to use the lowest possible dose of hydrocortisone to achieve optimal levels; taking a higher dose than needed can shut down production of cortisol by the adrenals. Your body will lower its production to some degree while you're supplementing but resume making higher levels when you stop.

Daily dosages of hydrocortisone vary from 10 to 40 mg for women and from 20 to 55 mg for men. Specific dosages and timing depend on the severity of your deficiency and when your shortfall occurs. Some doctors prescribe a larger dose in the morning and then lower doses as the day progresses, to mimic cortisol's natural circadian rhythm. Endocrine expert Thierry Hertoghe (2006) recommends the following dosing schedule.

	Severity of Deficiency	Hydrocortisone Dose
Women	Borderline	10 mg upon waking 5 mg at noon
	Mild	10 mg upon waking 10 mg at noon
	Moderate	15 mg upon waking 10 mg at noon 5 mg at 4 p.m.
	Severe	20 mg upon waking 10 mg at noon 5 mg at 4 p.m. 5 mg at bedtime
Men	Borderline	15 mg upon waking 5 mg at noon
	Mild	20 mg upon waking 10 mg at noon
	Moderate	25 mg upon waking 10 mg at noon 5 mg at 4 p.m.
	Severe	30 mg upon waking 10 mg at noon 10 mg at 4 p.m. 5 mg at bedtime

Dr. Hertoghe cautions that supplemental hydrocortisone can be harmful if you don't have sufficient levels of DHEA and sex hormones such as estrogen or testosterone to counter its effects. This imbalance can result in excessive tissue breakdown, leading to osteoporosis, decreased immune function, and thinning and bruising of skin. He recommends taking hydrocortisone only when necessary and using the smallest effective dose, while also correcting deficiencies of other hormones. If you don't respond well to hydrocortisone, Dr. Hertoghe recommends eating a more balanced diet and cutting out sweets to enhance the effectiveness of supplemental hydrocortisone (Hertoghe 2006).

Lastly, acute stress, such as surgery, an accident, or a severe illness or death in the family, can require you to take three to ten times your regular dose (Merke and Cutler 1997).

THE CONTROVERSY ABOUT HYDROCORTISONE VS. CORTISOL-LIKE PRODUCTS

Some physicians are reluctant to prescribe low-dose hydrocortisone, even if blood tests warrant it. This bias may stem from concern about known side effects of drugs like prednisone, prednisolone, and dexamethasone, which are chemically similar to cortisol. Prednisone is more than five times stronger than hydrocortisone and stays in the body much longer, and at daily doses over 5 mg, it can have serious side effects and even shut down your body's own cortisol production (Meikle and Tyler 1977).

However, doctors' reluctance to use low, physiologic doses of hydrocortisone may be lessening. Recent research has indicated that low-dose hydrocortisone can be successful in treating adrenal hyperplasia, rheumatoid arthritis (Hickling, Jacoby, and Kirwan 1998), sepsis (Klaitman and Almog 2003), and polymyalgia rheumatica, a systemic inflammatory disorder (Cutolo et al. 2002).

DHEA

The initial response to stress is an increase in levels of DHEA and cortisol (as well as adrenaline). Over time DHEA levels fall, followed by cortisol levels. Much less frequently, DHEA can remain high while cortisol drops first. UK hormone expert Dr. Durrant-Peatfield (2003) believes that this may indicate a problem with the body's ability to make cortisol from pregnenolone, and that it can be resolved only by taking hydrocortisone.

Deficiencies in male sex hormones, including DHEA, are fairly common in women as they age. Replacing deficient hormones can increase sex drive and muscle development. However, be aware that supplemental DHEA increases testosterone levels. If testosterone gets too high, women can experience masculinization, including increased facial hair, greasy face and hair, acne, strong body odor, menstrual irregularities, male-pattern hair loss, and clitoral enlargement. These effects are generally slow to develop and reversible when the dosage is reduced.

DHEA is available over the counter. You can find it in health food stores and online in capsules, liquid form, or transdermal cream, which can be rubbed into the skin. Typical dosages start at 5 mg per day for women and 25 mg for men. If tests have identified a significant deficiency, doses of 25 mg for women and 50 mg for men can substantially increase DHEA levels and are generally well tolerated.

Anyone using supplemental DHEA should have levels of DHEA-sulfate checked periodically. And, because DHEA can be converted to estrogen or testosterone, levels of these two hormones should be tested in both men and women. Some women report that DHEA supplementation causes symptoms of low estrogen (due to increase in the ratio of testosterone to estrogen), so watch for this side effect and others and adjust dosage levels as needed.

Benefits of supplemental DHEA are highly individual and hard to predict, even when levels are low. Many people benefit significantly, but others see no noticeable positive effects. Men with prostate disease should use DHEA with caution, as it can convert to testosterone or estrogen, which can cause excessive cell growth in the prostate.

PREGNENOLONE

Pregnenolone is a precursor to many adrenal hormones. Because of the numerous beneficial effects of this hormone, you should talk to your doctor about supplementing if your levels are low. It was used to treat arthritis for many years starting in the 1940s, so it has a long safety record. For arthritis, doses were up to 500 mg per day. A typical dose for raising levels is in the range of 10 to 50 mg per day, and doses up to 200 mg per day are generally considered safe. Be sure to have your levels tested after you start supplementing to make sure your dose is optimal.

Pregnenolone can be purchased over the counter at many health food stores or online. Work with your doctor to monitor your symptoms, pregnenolone levels, and levels of other hormones the body makes from pregnenolone to prevent symptoms of excess androgens, including acne and hair loss.

PROGESTERONE

Progesterone, made primarily in women's ovaries and men's testes, is a building block for other major hormones, including cortisol, DHEA, testosterone, and estrogen. If too much is used to produce cortisol, not enough is available to make testosterone or estrogen. Progesterone has an effect similar to licorice, inhibiting the enzyme that deactivates cortisol. As a result, it makes more cortisol available to your body. If your levels of progesterone are low, you can purchase low-dose progesterone skin cream over the counter. Stronger formulations are available by prescription in pill and cream form. A blood test can determine the right dosage for you, usually up to 20 mg for men and postmenopausal women and up to 200 mg for perimenopausal women who aren't ovulating.

ALDOSTERONE

If lab tests indicate you have severely depleted levels of aldosterone, talk to your doctor about supplementing with fludrocortisone (Florinef), a prescription drug with aldosterone-like effects, or, even better, with bioidentical aldosterone. The latter is available only through compound pharmacies, which specialize in making individualized hormone products. If you're only slightly deficient and don't require supplemental aldosterone, be sure to get enough salt in your diet to support electrolyte balance.

WHERE DOES THIS LEAVE US?

You've made a plan for trying acupuncture and taking vitamins, minerals, herbs, and other supplements to help balance hormone levels and support optimal adrenal function. You've worked with your doctor to test your levels of key hormones, whether you need to supplement any adrenal hormones, and what dosages and schedule are best for you.

The next step on your path to optimal adrenal function is to make sure your thyroid status isn't affecting your adrenals. The next chapter will give you all of the details you need on thyroid function and how it affects the adrenals, along with a symptom questionnaire, home tests and lab tests to assess thyroid function, and treatment options for hypothyroidism.

KEY POINTS

- Acupuncture can be helpful in normalizing cortisol levels by reducing excess cortisol production or supporting its production if your levels are low.

- To reduce the effects of high cortisol levels, try chromium, fish oil, magnesium, melatonin, phosphatidylserine, vitamin C, ashwagandha, *Ginkgo biloba*, ginseng, maca root, and *Rhodiola rosea*.

- To support adrenal function and boost levels of cortisol, try supplementing digestive enzymes, pantothenic acid, other B vitamins, sodium (from salt), vitamin C, ginseng, and licorice. Also be sure you're getting enough vitamin D—from sunshine, diet, or supplements.

- If your hormone levels are significantly low, work with your doctor to supplement with adrenal glandular extracts or bioidentical cortisol (hydrocortisone), DHEA, pregnenolone, progesterone, or aldosterone as needed. When taking supplemental hormones, be sure to have your levels tested periodically to make sure your dosage is right and that your levels aren't still too low or getting too high.

CHAPTER 6

Understanding the Relationship Between the Adrenals and the Thyroid

Your adrenals rely heavily on your thyroid to function correctly. None of the adrenals' vital activities can be accomplished without adequate thyroid support. In fact, virtually every cell in your body has receptors for both cortisol and thyroid hormones. You must have adequate levels of both in your cells for your body to do its job and be healthy.

If you have hypothyroidism (reduced thyroid function), production of cortisol and aldosterone drops. And conversely, if you have hyperthyroidism, or elevated thyroid activity, you produce higher levels of cortisol and aldosterone (Gordon and Southren 1977).

THE BASICS OF THYROID FUNCTION

Located at the base of the front of your neck, your thyroid gland is the engine for your metabolism, the process of turning food into energy. When your metabolism isn't working at full speed, everything in your body slows down. Every organ and gland, and even every cell, is affected, causing a general slowing of all physical and mental processes.

When your thyroid doesn't work properly, your body temperature is poorly regulated, so you'll have a hard time with heat and cold. Oxygen consumption is reduced, slowing down utilization of nutrients for energy. You're likely to be constipated and tired and experience weight gain and hair loss. Aches and pains develop, skin and hair dry out, and cholesterol levels rise. Impaired vision and hearing, sleeping disorders, numbness, and loss of libido are common. Worst of all are the mental and emotional problems: memory problems, cognitive slowdown, depression, rage, anxiety, and irritability.

Like your adrenals, your thyroid gland is regulated by your hypothalamus and pituitary glands. Your hypothalamus produces thyrotropin-releasing hormone (TRH), stimulating your pituitary to release thyroid-stimulating hormone (TSH). TSH triggers your thyroid to produce four hormones when needed: T1 (monoiodotyrosine), T2 (diiodotyrosine), T3 (triiodothyronine), and T4 (thyroxine).

The two thyroid hormones most critical to adrenal health are T3 and T4. Blood levels of T4 are approximately four times higher than levels of T3. However, you have relatively few T4 receptors and numerous T3 receptors, so T4 must be converted to T3 to have biological effect.

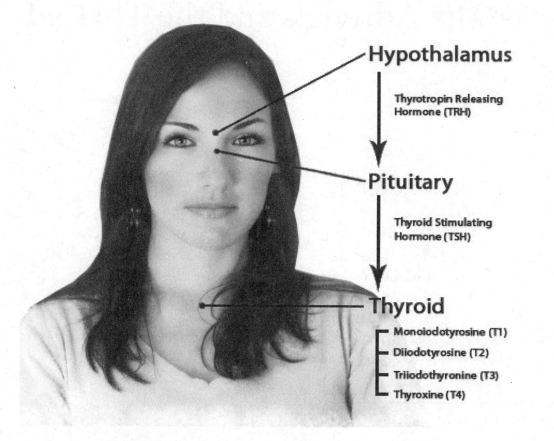

Thyroid stimulation pathway

Source: Kathryn Simpson, *The Women's Guide to Thyroid Health* (Oakland, CA: New Harbinger Publications, 2009).

THE CRITICAL RELATIONSHIP BETWEEN YOUR ADRENALS AND YOUR THYROID

Cortisol makes your thyroid work more efficiently, and thyroid hormones are vital for cortisol function. Optimum amounts of both cortisol and thyroid hormones—not too high and not too low—are important for normal thyroid and adrenal function.

Cortisol is necessary to produce thyroid hormones, and also necessary for your body to convert T4 to the active form T3, as well as for thyroid receptor function. When your thyroid hormone receptors aren't working properly, any thyroid hormones you do make can't get into your cells. Without enough cortisol, the thyroid receptors can eventually even disappear (until you correct the deficiency). Too much cortisol, on the other hand, causes thyroid resistance, where your tissues no longer respond to thyroid hormones as they should. Your levels of T3 and T4 will look normal, but you'll have symptoms of hypothyroidism.

Hypothyroidism slows your adrenal glands and also stresses your body, increasing adrenaline output and further taxing the adrenals. In addition, hypothyroidism leads to an increase in cortisol-binding globulin, a protein that binds cortisol and makes it unavailable to your body. You can see how vicious this cycle can become, with low thyroid function leading to low adrenal function, which leads to even lower thyroid function.

Hypothyroidism also causes a sluggish liver, preventing cortisol from being cleared from your body effectively. It builds up, giving you artificially high levels on lab tests. Once a thyroid deficiency is resolved, lab tests will reveal your true adrenal status.

What Is Reverse T3?

In order to actively affect your body, T4 must be converted into T3. Under normal conditions, a small amount of T3's inactive isomer (a mirror-image molecule), called reverse T3 (rT3), is formed in the process. Reverse T3 doesn't have any biological activity. It's designed as a brake, to slow down metabolism during starvation or famine, and some animals, such as bears, use it to slow their metabolism so they can hibernate through the winter without food (Demeneix and Henderson 1978).

When you're dieting or under a lot of stress and making high levels of cortisol in response to the situation, your body converts T4 to rT3 instead of T3. Reverse T3 ties up your thyroid receptors and prevents you from using the T3 you do have. This results in symptoms of hypothyroidism no matter what your actual levels of thyroid hormones are. That's why it's so hard to lose weight on an extreme diet. Your body thinks it's hibernating or starving and starts producing rT3 to get you through the long winter or famine.

EXERCISE: Hypothyroidism Symptom Evaluation

In order to optimize your adrenal function, it's important to determine whether hypothyroidism could be playing a part in your adrenal health. The first step in evaluating your thyroid function is to evaluate your symptoms. Note that, due to the close relationship between the thyroid and the adrenals, several of the symptoms of low thyroid function are similar to symptoms of deficient adrenal function. If the following questionnaire indicates that you may have hypothyroidism, try the simple home tests later in this chapter before you ask your doctor to test your levels of thyroid hormones. Armed with the results of these home tests, you can make a case for further evaluation.

In the following list, circle the number that most accurately reflects how each statement applies to you. The last fourteen statements have higher point values, reflecting that these symptoms indicate more serious or long-standing thyroid dysfunction. It's useful to fill out the questionnaire periodically so that you can assess your improvement, so you may want to make copies and leave this version blank.

0 = None or never   2 = Moderate or often

1 = Mild or occasionally   3 = Severe or always

At the bottom of each page, total up the points circled, then carry these totals forward to the end of the evaluation to get a total score.

0 1 2 3   I feel tired or fatigued.

0 1 2 3   I have weak or stiff knees.

0 1 2 3   My voice gets hoarse or weak.

0 1 2 3   I've been losing a lot of hair.

0 1 2 3   I don't perspire, no matter how hot it is or while I'm exercising.

0 1 2 3   I get strange sounds in my ears, such as ringing, buzzing, clicking, or rumbling, and/or experience temporary hearing impairment.

0 1 2 3   I have grooves on my fingernails, and/or they're soft and thin and crack and break easily.

0 1 2 3   I have aches and pains in my joints, hands, feet, back, and legs or between my shoulder blades.

0 1 2 3   I have nasal congestion and/or tend to get sinus infections.

0 1 2 3   I've started to talk more slowly and to have trouble enunciating.

0 1 2 3   I have a lot of tartar on my teeth.

Page total: _____

0   1   2   3   My tongue seems to be getting bigger; the sides are rippled from my teeth.

0   1   2   3   I'm not eating more but still gaining weight, and diet and exercise don't affect it.

0   1   2   3   My feet are getting flatter. I wear a larger shoe and/or my feet roll inward.

0   1   2   3   I tap my foot or jiggle my leg unconsciously.

0   1   2   3   I've had one or more miscarriages.

0   1   2   3   I tend to get ear infections.

0   1   2   3   I have a buildup of earwax.

0   1   2   3   I clench or grind my teeth, especially at night.

0   1   2   3   I have poor night vision.

0   1   2   3   I've have TMJ syndrome (temporomandibular joint syndrome).

0   1   2   3   I have fungal infections of my toes and/or ingrown toenails.

0   1   2   3   My lips look swollen.

0   1   2   3   The skin on my legs is rough and/or scaly, particularly below my knees.

0   1   2   3   My face and/or lips are pale.

0   1   2   3   My hair is becoming fine, dry, and brittle.

0   1   2   3   I have moles and warts.

0   1   2   3   I have dental problems, including lots of cavities.

0   1   2   3   I tend to get irritable.

0   1   2   3   My hair is prematurely gray.

0   1   2   3   My hands and feet get pins-and-needles feelings.

0   1   2   3   I have a hard time concentrating.

0   1   2   3   I seem to get sick more and illnesses linger longer than they used to.

0   1   2   3   My skin is puffy looking; even my back looks puffy.

0   1   2   3   I have a hard time falling asleep at night.

Page total: _____

0   1   2   3   The skin on my upper arms and thighs feels thick when I pinch it.

0   1   2   3   My skin and/or the whites of my eyes are yellowish.

0   1   2   3   I sometimes have heart palpitations and skipped heartbeats.

0   1   2   3   I feel tired even if I get a lot of sleep and/or rest.

0   1   2   3   I have lost a lot of my body hair.

0   1   2   3   Heat and/or cold bothers me.

0   1   2   3   I tend to get urinary tract or bladder infections.

0   1   2   3   I have a weak, slow pulse.

0   1   2   3   My hands and feet feel cold.

0   1   2   3   I have a hard time catching my breath.

0   1   2   3   I have strange dreams or nightmares.

0   1   2   3   I've choked on small objects or have choking sensations.

0   1   2   3   I have dry skin.

0   1   2   3   My fingernail beds are pale.

0   1   2   3   I yawn a lot even when I'm not tired.

For the rest of the questions, circle 0 for no or the number on the right for yes.

0   10   I've had infertility problems.

0   10   I have fibrocystic breasts.

0   10   I'm chronically constipated.

0   10   My neck is thickening or bulging in the front under my Adam's apple.

0   15   The outside ends of my eyebrows are getting much thinner and shorter.

0   15   I have psoriasis, eczema, vitiligo, or red, flaky skin on my face.

0   15   I have Raynaud's syndrome.

0   20   My heart appears enlarged on an X-ray.

0   20   I have a chronically low basal body temperature.

Page total: _____

0   20   I have gout.

0   20   I have carpal tunnel syndrome.

0   20   I have fibromyalgia.

0   20   I have an autoimmune disease.

0   20   I have ADD (attention deficit disorder).

Page total: _____

Total Score: _____

Interpreting Your Results

Scores between 8 and 12 indicate early signs of hypothyroidism and metabolic slowing. Scores between 13 and 20 indicate a good likelihood of hypothyroidism. Scores over 20 indicate significant thyroid function deficiency (and probably an adrenal imbalance).

With any of these results, have a complete physical, including a thyroid exam and lab tests for free T3, free T4, TSH, and reverse T3 levels, as well as thyroid antibodies if your doctor feels it's warranted. Once you start taking steps to address any thyroid hormone problems, complete this symptom questionnaire every three months until all of your symptoms are gone. You may be surprised at how quickly many of them resolve.

THYROID TESTING RECOMMENDATIONS

If your symptom evaluation indicates that you may have hypothyroidism, your next step is to do the following self-tests, which will give you additional information about your thyroid status and help persuade your doctor to order blood tests.

Self-Tests You Can Do at Home

The following tests are easy to do and require only a basal thermometer and an inexpensive bottle of iodine.

IODINE DEFICIENCY TEST

Iodine is essential for your thyroid gland to produce thyroid hormones. Lack of iodine in your diet decreases thyroid hormone production and conversion of T4 to T3, which can lead to hypothyroidism. Try this test to see if an iodine deficiency might be causing or exacerbating your thyroid problem.

1. Buy 2 percent tincture of iodine at the drugstore.

2. Use the applicator to apply a patch of iodine the size of a quarter on your stomach or thigh.

3. Observe the spot for twenty-four hours. If it disappears in less than twenty-four hours, it indicates iodine deficiency. The faster it disappears, the greater the deficiency.

If you don't use much salt, or use non-iodized salt, you may be deficient in iodine. If so, you can either use more iodized salt or take an iodine supplement.

PINCH TEST

A simple pinch test can indicate whether you have myxedema, a symptom of low thyroid function. Myxedema, caused by a buildup of waste in the tissues, results in swelling and causes tissues to adhere to the skin. It's most commonly seen in the face (around the eyes and on the jawline) and the front of the upper arms and legs.

Pinch a fold of skin on your upper arm between your thumb and forefinger. If the skin feels thick and you can't pinch a small amount of it, you may have myxedema.

BASAL BODY TEMPERATURE TEST

Basal body temperature (or the temperature of the body at rest) is a reliable indicator of metabolic rate. If your thyroid is healthy, you'll generally have a consistent basal body temperature near 98.4°F. If your temperature is below 97.8°F, it's an indicator of low thyroid function. Higher than normal readings could indicate a low-grade infection, which you might want to consider following up on.

Most doctors recommend that you track your temperature for ten days in a row. Women who still menstruate should start testing on day 1 of their period; others can do it anytime. Get a basal thermometer, which is more sensitive and accurate than a regular thermometer.

1. When you awake in the morning, remain in bed and put the thermometer under your arm or tongue.

2. Lie still for ten minutes.

3. Remove the thermometer, read it, and write down your results.

Thyroid Lab Tests

If you have symptoms of low thyroid function or positive home tests, make an appointment with your doctor to get your levels of thyroid hormones tested, including TSH, free T4 and T3, and reverse T3. It's important to look at *free* T3 and T4, not total amounts, because these reflect the amount of thyroid hormones available to your cells.

Thyroid antibody tests for thyroid peroxidase antibodies (TPOAb), thyroglobulin antibodies (TgAb), and thyrotropin receptor antibodies (TRAb) are also valuable in detecting autoimmune conditions that cause hypothyroidism. If you have any of these antibodies, your doctor may want to start you on thyroid hormone therapy, which can sometimes stop the autoimmune activity and the damage to your thyroid gland.

TSH TESTING

The first test most doctors do for hypothyroidism is measuring levels of TSH. TSH levels rise to stimulate production of thyroid hormones when their levels fall, so elevated TSH indicates that you have hypothyroidism.

Unfortunately this test can't always accurately diagnose hypothyroidism without additional tests, for several reasons:

- Laboratory reference ranges are only guidelines, and many people function best with higher levels of thyroid hormones.

- Many large testing labs use outdated TSH reference ranges. Many thyroid specialists, including Dr. Thierry Hertoghe, recommend that anyone with a TSH level over 2.5 mIU/ml be treated for hypothyroidism. (Remember, the higher your TSH level, the more impaired your thyroid function is.) Old ranges still being used go up to 5 or even 7 mIU/ml. When doctors rely on these outdated ranges, they misdiagnose patients with hypothyroidism as having normal thyroid function.

- If you have a problem with the glands that regulate the thyroid—the pituitary or hypothalamus—your pituitary may not increase production of TSH even when thyroid hormone levels are low. This condition is called central hypothyroidism.

- Resistance to thyroid hormones can be caused by substances either made by the body, such as antibodies or excessive cortisol, or from external sources, such as toxins. This cause of hypothyroidism may be more common than many others, and it may not be detected by TSH tests.

Despite these drawbacks, blood levels of TSH are still useful, as this test diagnoses primary hypothyroidism accurately if the right ranges are used. (Primary hypothyroidism is a problem with the thyroid itself, as opposed to the glands that regulate its function.) It's also useful to track TSH levels over time, just like cholesterol levels and results of other routine tests, to monitor changes in your thyroid function.

T3 AND T4 TESTING

It's important to measure levels of free T3 and T4 to see if they're low, and to determine whether you're converting enough T4 to T3. If you have a low T3 level, when taking supplemental thyroid hormones you may need either a combination product with T3 and T4, such as a glandular product, or a T3 drug combined with a T4 drug.

REVERSE T3 TESTING

The rT3 test detects if you're converting too much T4 to rT3. If your lab results show normal TSH and low, normal, or even elevated T3 and T4 levels, but elevated rT3, you may benefit from thyroid hormone therapy. The right medication is vital to correcting this problem. Taking biologically active T3 will help displace rT3, whereas more T4 can convert to more rT3. So your thyroid medications should contain some T3.

TREATING LOW THYROID FUNCTION

If you have just a few symptoms of low thyroid function or your TSH is climbing but you're not in the hypothyroid range yet, try supporting your thyroid function with optimal diet and the vitamins, minerals, and supplements discussed below to see if you can increase your thyroid function. I've included generally recommended dosages, but you should work with your doctor or nutritionist to determine the doses appropriate for you.

Vitamins, Minerals, and Herbs

With the modifications to your diet discussed in chapter 7 or the addition of over-the-counter supplements, you can do a great deal to support your thyroid. All of the nutrients and supplements discussed below can be helpful, but iodine and tyrosine are especially important, as these two building blocks are needed to make and utilize thyroid hormones.

Ashwagandha. Ashwagandha improves thyroid function by increasing levels of T3 and T4 (Panda and Kar 1998). The generally recommended dose is 250 mg per day.

B Vitamins. B vitamins play an important role in the manufacture of thyroid hormones and their uptake into cells. Good food sources of B vitamins are brewer's yeast, almonds, wheat germ, wild rice, mushrooms, egg yolks, rice bran, wheat bran, peanuts, liver, poultry (white meat), sunflower seeds, tuna, salmon, trout, beans, walnuts, brown rice, and bananas. Supplements containing a combination of the primary B vitamins will be labeled "B complex."

Coleus forskohlii. This herb, used widely in Ayurvedic medicine, has been shown to increase the production of thyroid hormones and stimulate their release (Haye et al. 1985). The generally recommended dose is 10 to 50 mg per day.

Guggul. Guggul (*Commiphora mukul*) has strong thyroid stimulating actions that increase iodine uptake and levels of T3 (Panda and Kar 1999). The generally recommended dose is 25 mg once or twice per day.

Iodine. If you have only slightly low thyroid function, it's sometimes possible to restore thyroid health with adequate iodine supplementation. Good food sources of iodine include eggs, fish, seafood, sea vegetables, yogurt, milk, and strawberries. Iodine is added to table salt in the United States, and just over ½ teaspoon of iodized salt provides the recommended daily iodine allowance of 150 mcg. You can also take an iodine supplement if you aren't getting enough through diet.

Selenium. Selenium plays an important role in regulating T3 and T4 thyroid hormone activity. Food sources of selenium include cereal grains (wheat, rice, and so on), nuts (Brazil nuts and walnuts), legumes (soybeans), animal products (eggs, beef, chicken, and cheese), and seafood (tuna) The generally recommended dose is 100 mcg per day.

Tyrosine. Your thyroid combines the amino acid tyrosine with iodine and then converts it to T4, which is then converted to T3. Food sources of tyrosine include wheat, oats, dairy products, chicken, fish, pork, avocados, bananas, lima beans, almonds, and sesame seeds. Tyrosine supplements are also available. The generally recommended dose is about 1,000 mg per day. Be cautious about taking high doses. All amino acids can be toxic at high levels, and supplementing individual amino acids can also create imbalances with other amino acids.

Vitamin A. Vitamin A is involved in the uptake of iodine into your thyroid gland. A deficiency can also reduce production of TSH by the pituitary. Food sources of vitamin A and its precursor, beta-carotene, include kale, sweet potatoes, lettuce, carrots, winter squash, pumpkin, spinach, cantaloupe, broccoli, asparagus, and liver. The generally recommended dose is 2,500 IU of vitamin A per day; an equivalent amount of beta-carotene would be about 8,500 IU.

Vitamin C. Vitamin C improves oral absorption of T4 drugs. Good food sources include guavas, peppers, citrus, strawberries, broccoli, cauliflower, brussels sprouts, papaya, parsley, kale, and other leafy greens, including turnip, collard, and mustard greens. The generally recommended dose is 1,000 to 3,000 mg per day.

Zinc. This trace mineral is important for thyroid function, including conversion of T4 to T3. Food sources of zinc include split peas, whole grains, sunflower seeds, pecans, Brazil nuts, almonds, walnuts, ginger root, maple syrup, oysters, sardines, beef, lamb, and turkey. The generally recommended dose is 15 mg per day, plus 500 mcg of copper.

Thyroid Medication Treatment Options

If you're diagnosed with hypothyroidism, you'll need to take supplemental thyroid hormones. Your doctor may initially have you take a T4-only drug, such as Synthroid, Levothroid, or Levoxyl, all brand names for levothyroxine.

Treating hypothyroidism with a T4-only drug is the current standard-of-care practice, which means what most doctors would do under the circumstances. Some people do fine on this treatment, but if you can't convert T4 to T3 effectively, have low levels of T3 or excess rT3, or don't experience complete resolution of symptoms on T4, talk to your doctor about adding T3. Clinical studies show that many people on thyroid hormone therapy feel better with both T3 and T4 (Bunevicius et al. 1999).

Combination therapies make use of both the T3 drug liothyronine (Cytomel) and a T4 drug. Glandular products, made of desiccated pig thyroid gland, have all the hormones the thyroid gland produces: T1, T2, T3, and T4. Brand names include Armour, Westhroid, and Nature-throid; you can also obtain glandular thyroid products from compound pharmacies. There have been significant quality issues with these products over the last two years, so until this situation is resolved, you may have to try a combination of synthetic T3 and T4 drugs.

Successfully treating hypothyroidism with supplemental thyroid hormones will probably involve some trial and error to find your optimal drug and dose. You may have to try different products or combinations of products, as well as different dosing schedules to determine your optimal treatment regime. The best approach is to increase your dose in small increments, to increase your metabolism slowly and gently.

Doctors usually start at a very low dose. If the dose is high enough for you, you should notice a change soon, with symptoms subsiding and an increased sense of well-being. If this fades after a couple of days or weeks, don't get discouraged. It generally means that your metabolism has increased and you need a higher dose to sustain this new level. Work with your doctor to find the dose where your symptoms don't return.

THYROID THERAPY WITH WEAK ADRENALS

Resolving hypothyroidism when you have adrenal fatigue is more complex than if your adrenal health is robust. When you take thyroid medication, your metabolism speeds up, and if you have insufficient adrenal function, your body can't increase cortisol production fast enough to meet the demand. So you may feel worse instead of better—until you resolve the situation.

There are clear signals of this situation if you know what to look for. If you start taking thyroid medication and it either doesn't seem to work at all or you have symptoms of hyperthyroidism with very low levels of medication (trembling hands, insomnia, feeling unusually hot, being irritable, and so on), you probably have low adrenal function. If you don't adequately treat any adrenal insufficiency, it's incredibly difficult to successfully treat hypothyroidism.

ᚷ *My Story*

When I first started taking supplemental thyroid hormones, I thought I'd finally regained my health. All of my symptoms were gone, and I felt great for two weeks. Unfortunately, just when I thought I was finally completely well, my symptoms started coming back.

Once again, I was exhausted in the afternoons. The brain fog and insomnia returned, as well as the bladder, vision, and other problems. Although discouraged, I was heartened by the fact that I'd been completely symptom free just the week before. I started researching and came across the connection between thyroid and adrenal function. What I read made me think that my adrenals were exhausted and not making adequate cortisol.

Sure enough, cortisol testing showed extremely low levels throughout the day. I started taking bioidentical cortisol (hydrocortisone) four times a day (for a total of 25 mg per day) and soon felt completely well again.

WHERE DOES THIS LEAVE US?

You now have the tools you need to understand the complex and intertwined relationship between your thyroid and adrenal glands. The symptom evaluation and simple home tests you completed have given you a clearer sense of how your thyroid is functioning and whether or not it's playing a part in your adrenal fatigue. If your thyroid seems to be involved, now you can start working on solutions. Schedule an appointment with your doctor to share the valuable symptom information you've gathered, and to have lab tests to assess your thyroid function.

In the next chapter, we'll take a look at the cornerstone of any sound wellness program: diet. I'll help you make sure that you're eating foods that will stabilize and support your adrenal hormone levels, and we'll also take a look at other issues related to diet, like when and how much you eat, and foods and other substances to be avoided.

KEY POINTS

🐾 Your adrenals and thyroid have a vital reciprocal relationship. Cortisol makes your thyroid hormones work more efficiently and vice versa. Hypothyroidism slows the adrenals' output of hormones.

🐾 Cortisol is necessary to produce thyroid hormones, for your body to convert T4 to the active form T3, and for thyroid receptor function.

🐾 Excess cortisol causes thyroid resistance, where your tissues no longer respond to thyroid hormones as they should, resulting in symptoms of hypothyroidism.

🐾 Stress causes high levels of cortisol and conversion of T4 to reverse T3 instead of T3.

🐾 Hypothyroidism causes metabolic slowdown, with ill effects on blood pressure, body temperature, fluid balance, digestion, elimination, heart and nerve health, breathing, liver function, mobility, sleep, and energy levels. It can also cause widespread pain and stiffness, compromised immune function, and problems with everything from hair, skin, nails, and teeth to weight and muscular function to cognitive function and emotional balance.

🐾 Home tests for thyroid function include the iodine deficiency test, the pinch test, and the basal body temperature test.

🐾 Initial thyroid lab tests should include levels of TSH, free T3, free T4, and reverse T3.

🐾 Supplements and herbs that have been shown to support thyroid function are ashwagandha, B vitamins, *Coleus forskohlii*, guggul, iodine, tyrosine, selenium, vitamin A, vitamin C, and zinc.

🐾 You will need to take thyroid medication if you have hypothyroidism. This may mean taking only T4, only T3, or a combination of T4 and T3, depending on your lab results and your response to therapy.

CHAPTER 7

Eating for Adrenal Health

One of the most important things you can do to support your adrenal glands is to eat a balanced diet that will help control your blood sugar levels, insulin production, and cortisol levels. Our transition from the hunter-gatherer diet eaten by human beings for more than two million years to modern, processed foods has had a profound effect on our adrenals. This change has occurred far too rapidly for our bodies to adapt to this new way of eating—if they ever do! Our current diet has far more inflammatory effects due to a different mix of fatty acids and the abundance of refined carbs, sugars, and foods containing common allergens like wheat, dairy, and soy.

Fortunately, it's easy to turn this situation around by adopting an anti-inflammatory diet. This doesn't mean that you have to follow a complicated diet plan or start eating special foods. It simply requires you to eat good-quality protein, fats, and complex carbohydrates at every meal. This will help keep your blood sugar levels more stable, putting less strain on your adrenals. It will also help you lose that stubborn abdominal weight often associated with both elevated cortisol and subsequent low cortisol.

When you eat and how much you eat matters too. If you're already eating a variety of healthy foods, you may simply need to adjust when you eat or portion sizes to keep blood sugar, insulin, and cortisol—and calories—under control.

WHEN TO EAT

Eat smaller, more frequent meals, and don't skip meals. It isn't unreasonable, or unnatural, to eat five to six times a day. When you go too long between meals, your body releases more cortisol. This stimulates your appetite and causes cravings.

Eat breakfast within an hour of when you wake up, and have a good snack within two to three hours to forestall blood sugar swings and cravings. Breakfast establishes our blood sugar foundation for the entire day, and we're programmed to digest a lot of calories early in the day. Without a balanced meal, your blood sugar starts a roller-coaster ride that can exhaust you by day's end. For a balance of fats, protein, and complex carbs, consider having two eggs, bacon, and cooked whole-grain cereal.

Having a balanced snack in the midmorning will help you resist the mochas and croissants on the coffee cart or toaster pastries in your pantry. Try to incorporate fat, protein, and complex carbs into your snacks. This could be unsweetened Greek yogurt with fruit and nuts, cheese and whole-grain crackers, celery and nut butter, or bean dip and whole-grain tortilla chips.

Keep this pattern going throughout the day. Having eaten so well in the morning, you may find that you can have a lighter lunch. For most of us, blood sugar gets low around 3 p.m. So in the midafternoon, you may find yourself getting tired and having difficulty concentrating. Turning to caffeine or sugar to give yourself quick energy can backfire, as your blood sugar spikes and then drops. Instead, have another balanced snack to tide you over until dinnertime.

Having a small, balanced evening snack can help regulate your blood sugar throughout the night. Try a taco made with a corn tortilla, brown rice, beans, and salsa made with olive oil. The combination of beans with grains, nuts, or seeds creates a whole protein, containing all of the essential amino acids. Another easy adrenal-friendly evening snack is bean soup. Beans are a good source of both soluble and insoluble dietary fiber, which prevents blood sugar levels from increasing quickly after a meal (Jenkins et al. 1980). They're also full of B vitamins, which can help protect your heart from the effects of elevated cortisol. Avoid high-sugar foods after dinner so your blood sugar doesn't spike and keep you awake, and then plummet in the middle of the night, which will cause a cortisol surge. This can interfere with growth hormone production, and possibly disrupt your sleep.

HOW MUCH TO EAT

According to the U.S. Department of Agriculture (2002), the U.S. population is consuming more food—to the tune of several hundred more calories per person per day—than in 1985. But even though portion sizes are bigger, many of us aren't getting proper nutrition. The increase in calorie consumption between 1985 and 2000 consisted of grains (mainly refined grains), up 46 percent; fats, up 24 percent; and sugars, up 23 percent. Fruits and vegetables increased by only 8 percent, and meat and dairy together declined by 1 percent (Putnam, Allshouse, and Kantor 2002). Unfortunately, sugar and refined carbs are empty calories—devoid of important nutrients. For most people this consumption of more food or higher-calorie foods isn't balanced by an increase in physical activity (Putnam, Allshouse, and Kantor 2002). In addition, more calories result in higher cortisol levels.

WHAT TO EAT

One simple rule to follow is to eat foods as they're found in nature. If you apply this principle as often as possible, it's hard to get in trouble. After all, sodas and fast food can't be harvested from the fields. As mentioned, every meal should include a balance of good-quality proteins, fats, and complex carbohydrates. A good rule of thumb is to eat the same amount of calories of protein and complex carbs and slightly fewer calories from fat. Overall, approximately 37 percent of your diet should be protein, 37 percent should be complex carbs, and the remaining 26 percent should be fat.

An example of a perfectly balanced meal is a grilled steak, pork chop, or chicken breast; brown rice or another whole grain with butter; broccoli or other nonstarchy vegetables; and a salad dressed with olive oil and lemon juice. Try eating like this for a week and see how you feel. It should noticeably reduce your food cravings. Once you experience how good you feel when you eat more healthfully, it will become easier to balance your diet.

Carbohydrates

Carbohydrates consist of sugar molecules. Simple carbohydrates, or monosaccharides, are single sugar molecules; oligosaccharides consist of short chains of sugar molecules; and polysaccharides consist of longer chains—what we usually think of as complex carbohydrates. While these distinctions are important, any of the three can be healthful if eaten in moderation and from whole food sources.

The more important distinction is between refined grains and whole grains. When grains are refined, their fiber-rich outer shell is removed, and often the nutrient-dense germ is removed as well. Brown rice becomes white rice, whole wheat flour becomes white flour, and so on, with the end result that, robbed of their fiber, they convert to blood sugar much more quickly than whole grains do. And because many of their nutrients have been removed, your body has to use stored nutrients to extract energy from these processed grains.

Besides whole grains, vegetables and beans are also rich in complex carbohydrates, including fiber. Fiber adds bulk that causes food to be converted to blood sugar more slowly, resulting in a slower release of insulin, and in lesser quantities. This is important because the amount of insulin we make determines whether food is stored as fat or burned for energy.

All carbs other than indigestible fiber eventually become blood sugar, which is what supplies energy to the brain and the rest of the body. In fact, the brain depends entirely on glucose, or blood sugar, for energy. So carbs can be a good thing—in the right quantities and forms. It's only when we eat too many carbs or too many refined carbs that the excess gets stored as fat. So it's important to restrict refined carbs but at the same time to eat enough complex carbs. This means cutting back on anything with white flour or sugar: cake, cookies, donuts, bread, pastry, cereals, pasta, soft drinks, and even fruit juices. Always choose whole-grain versions of bread, pasta, tortillas, cereals, and other grain-based foods.

SUGAR

In 2004, average sugar consumption in the United States was more than 22 teaspoons of sugar a day (Johnson et al. 2009). It's in everything from soft drinks to salad dressing. No matter what the source, there has been a staggering increase in recent centuries. In the 1900s, annual sugar consumption averaged about 90 pounds per person; in the 1800s it was around 18 pounds; and in the 1700s a mere 4 pounds (Johnson and Gower 2009).

Sugar is devoid of any nutritional value beyond the calories it provides for energy, so processing it puts the same demands on your body as refined carbs do: Your body must use its own stores of vitamins and minerals to metabolize refined sugar.

We're also eating the wrong type of sugar. Many food and drink manufacturers use high-fructose corn syrup in their products. Your body metabolizes fructose differently than glucose. It's much harder on your liver and increases production of uric acid, which raises blood pressure and can damage your kidneys as well as increase the risk of gout (Johnson and Gower 2009).

Generations past ate their sweets with their meals—a smart practice, because as long as you eat sweets (in moderation!) with a balanced meal, your blood sugar won't be too adversely affected. The total amount of carbs you eat—and how well-balanced your diet is overall, is as important as the type of carbs consumed. So if you'd like a piece of cake now and then, just substitute those calories for other carbohydrates in your meal, like bread or pasta. For instance, if your dinner consists of a fish fillet, salad, a baked potato, and a corn muffin, you could have a cookie instead of the muffin. When you do indulge, try to eat sweets made with whole grains, like an oatmeal cookie or a slice of whole-grain cake, rather than sugar-based sweets like candy or baked goods made with refined grains.

As an interesting side note, be aware that many foods marketed as low-fat are full of refined sugar, which is added to enhance taste. So people who think they're doing themselves a favor by eating these supposedly preferable low-fat alternatives are often eating much more sugar than they realize.

COMPLEX CARBOHYDRATES

Complex carbohydrates and whole grains have many health benefits. Complex carbs help regulate blood sugar by releasing their sugars more slowly; think of them as sustained-release fuel for your brain and body. They also help you feel full longer after eating.

Carbohydrate-rich whole foods, such as fruits, vegetables, whole grains, and legumes, are also high in fiber. Fiber comes in two forms: soluble and insoluble. Because soluble fiber attracts water and turns into a gel during digestion, it traps other carbohydrates, which also acts to slow the release of blood sugar and prevent insulin surges. As a result, high-fiber foods give you longer-lasting energy than refined and simple carbs do. They also tend to be low in fat and calories and rich in antioxidants, vitamins, and other nutrients. They've been proven to lower cholesterol and prevent, or even reverse, conditions like constipation, heart disease, colon and rectal cancer, diverticulosis, breast cancer, diabetes, and obesity (Galisteo, Duarte, and Zarzuelo 2008).

In addition, eating high-fiber foods can help you lose weight. They require you to chew longer, so you eat more slowly and your body has more time to feel full. Therefore, you're less likely to overeat. And when you consume high-fiber food, you'll feel full after consuming fewer calories.

Whole grains and products made from them are a good source of complex carbohydrates, as are fresh fruits and vegetables. Try to eat lots of different brightly colored fruits and vegetables every day: sweet potatoes, beets, carrots, bell peppers, broccoli, berries, citrus fruits, and dark leafy green vegetables, such as spinach and kale. Different colors of produce contain different nutrients, so by eating a rainbow of colors you'll get the widest range of nutrients to support your adrenals.

Choose organic fruits and vegetables whenever possible. Organic food is grown and produced without synthetic fertilizers, pesticides, or use of sewer sludge (which contains substances such as disinfectant or cleaning products—whatever people put down the drain). In addition, they aren't genetically modified and haven't been irradiated or treated with hormones or antibiotics. These chemicals and modified foods can be stressors for the body and therefore have the potential to cause increased production of cortisol. People with adrenal fatigue tend to have chemical sensitivities, and what little adrenal function they have left can be further depleted by exposure to toxins, including the chemicals used on commercially grown produce.

Fats

Dietary fats are necessary for many critical physiological functions, including manufacturing hormones. Cholesterol, that much-maligned substance, is used to make steroid hormones. If you don't have enough cholesterol, you may find your levels of both adrenal and sex hormones dropping.

Beginning in the 1960s, the American Heart Association (1961) and others recommended substituting carbohydrates for fat to reduce bad cholesterol. Sadly, high-carbohydrate diets have now been shown to increase bad cholesterol and decrease good cholesterol (Frost et al. 1999). Though well-intentioned, the earlier recommendation has resulted in increased incidence of heart disease, as well as diabetes and other inflammatory conditions and lowered hormone levels.

When it comes to fat, both quantity and quality are important. For optimum health, your body needs all three major categories of fat: saturated fats, such as butter, coconut oil, palm oil, and lard; unsaturated fats, such as safflower and corn oil; and monounsaturated fats from nuts, seeds, and olives and their oils, and canola oil.

Instead of restricting all fats, eat healthy fats and don't feel guilty about it. After all, the typical Eskimo or Inuit daily diet is over 50 percent fat, and it keeps them healthy year-round (Gadsby 2004). One theory suggests that it's because the cold-water fish and sea mammals they eat are rich in essential fatty acids, primarily omega-3s. Eskimos maintain a healthy weight eating this high-fat diet, but as soon as they start eating refined and simple carbs, they get fat. For those consuming the traditional high-fat diet of the far north, the death rate from heart disease is about half that of the U.S. population.

Fats slow the digestive process and help control blood sugar levels. Because they take so long to digest, they keep you from getting hungry for a longer time than carbohydrates. Each gram of fat provides 9 calories of energy for your body, compared with 4 calories per gram of carbohydrates or protein. Fats are also necessary for assimilating fat-soluble vitamins from food or supplements. If you're taking fat-soluble vitamins like A, D, E, or K, always take them with a fat to facilitate absorption.

OMEGA-3 AND OMEGA-6 FATTY ACIDS

Omega-3 and omega-6 fatty acids are both necessary for good health and controlling inflammation (Simopoulos 2002). Each comes in several varieties. Two of them—linoleic acid (an omega-6) and alpha-linolenic acid (an omega-3) must be obtained from the diet, as the body can't manufacture them. Strictly speaking, these are the only two essential fatty acids (EFAs), since your body can manufacture other omega-3s and omega-6s from these building blocks. However, the popular term for all omega-3s and omega-6s is "essential fatty acids," so I'll use the term that way here.

EFAs constitute 70 percent of your brain and nerve tissue and are vital for their functioning. They're also critical for adrenal and thyroid function and in manufacturing hormones. In addition to needing an adequate amount of EFAs, you need to keep an eye on the ratio between omega-6s and omega-3s. Our bodies function best with about a two to one ratio of omega-6s to omega-3s. But in the United States, most people eat twenty to thirty times more omega-6s than omega-3s.

If you have too much omega-6 in your diet, your cells can't use omega-3 effectively. This imbalance can lead to increased inflammation and exacerbation of all the conditions inflammation creates, such as allergic and degenerative disorders. On the other hand, there's a wealth of research on the beneficial effects of omega-3s in preventing and even reversing chronic diseases like cancer, cardiovascular disease, and inflammatory and autoimmune diseases (Simopoulos 2002).

Foods high in omega-3s include sardines, salmon, walnuts, flaxseeds, and dark green vegetables. Omega-6s are found in higher amounts in vegetable oils such as soybean, corn, safflower, and sunflower. They're also abundant in meat from grain-fed livestock.

One important note in regard to all oils: They are sensitive to heat, and some, like soy, canola, sunflower, and corn oil, become harmful when heated (Grootveld et al. 2001). Oils are also sensitive to light and exposure to oxygen, so keep them in a cool, dry place or the refrigerator.

SATURATED FATS

Dietary saturated fat is necessary for the production of cortisol. It's high in cholesterol, the precursor for adrenal hormones. We actually make most of our cholesterol, but we also need to get some from eating saturated fats, which are primarily found in animal products. Fat occurring naturally in animal tissues contains varying proportions of saturated and unsaturated fat. Some of the health problems associated with consuming animal products appear to be dependent on what the animals eat, as this determines the composition of their fats (Weill, Chesneau, and Safraou 2002).

Foods containing a high proportion of saturated fat include dairy products (cream, cheese, and butter); fatty meats and lard; and coconut oil and palm kernel oil. A word of caution: Don't take this advice as granting free license to consume too much saturated fat. It's important to eat it in moderation. The Nutrition Facts panel on most packaged foods gives a good guideline: Aim for less than 20 to 25 grams of saturated fat daily.

Grain-Fed vs. Free-Range Animal Products

Mass production of poultry, meat, eggs, and dairy products has taken over from small, family-owned farms. It's more profitable and prices can be lower. However, it comes at a cost to nutrition as well as adrenal health.

Free-range chicken, cattle, pigs, and sheep eat plants, which are typically relatively rich in omega-3 fatty acids, and wild fish eat algae or smaller fish that eat algae, also relatively rich in omega-3s. Modern, conventionally raised animals, however, eat grain—even the fish eat soy pellets. Grains and soy are higher in omega-6s, and therefore meat from animals or fish raised on these foods is higher in omega-6s as well. So the best sources of animal protein are wild or free-range animals (George and Bhopal 1995).

Animals raised on grain also have lower nutritional value and more total fat. Their meat contains less vitamin E, beta-carotene, and vitamin C (Nilzén et al. 2001). Meat from free-range animals, on the other hand, has less saturated fat and more polyunsaturated and monounsaturated fat (Hoffman 2006). Organic eggs from hens that eat a diet of insects and green plants often have a three to one ratio of omega-6s to omega-3s, whereas eggs from farmed hens can contain as much as nineteen times more omega-6 than omega-3 (Simopoulos and Salem 1992).

Another little known benefit of a natural diet of grasses for cows is that when they eat foods high in omega-3s, they have 30 to 40 percent lower methane emissions. Believe it or not, the burps that cows release while digesting foods low in omega-3s cause 5 to 10 percent of greenhouse gas emissions in this country (Smith et al. 2007).

Interestingly, grain-fed cows are now suffering from the same maladies that humans are. Many are insulin resistant due to their diet, and from being raised in crowded, stressful conditions, which causes them to binge eat (Mason 2010).

TRANS OR HYDROGENATED FATS

The processed fats known as *trans fats* should be avoided at all costs. These more shelf-stable fats were created over one hundred years ago when refrigeration wasn't universally available. To make them, polyunsaturated fats are hydrogenated, meaning hydrogen is added to give them a molecular structure similar to saturated fats. This helps prevent spoilage; that's why most candy bars and so many other processed foods last over a year instead of just weeks. Hydrogenated and partially hydrogenated oils raise levels of bad cholesterol (LDL), lower good cholesterol (HDL), interfere with cellular function, and block the body's use of important healthful fats.

Trans fats are widely used in processed food because they're cheaper and have a longer shelf life. They're also used in restaurants for frying because they can be reused longer. They've been banned in several U.S. cities and counties and in California, but packaged foods are exempt, so keep reading labels!

Protein

Adequate protein is necessary to build, repair, and maintain your entire body. Proteins are made up of different combinations of amino acids, which fall into two categories: essential and nonessential. Our bodies can make nonessential amino acids, but essential amino acids must come from the foods we eat.

The term "complete protein" refers to foods that have all eight essential amino acids in balanced amounts. Most animal foods offer complete protein, but only relatively few plant foods do, such as amaranth, buckwheat, quinoa. Soy also provides complete protein, but should be used sparingly (discussed below). Most plant foods are low in or completely lacking one or more essential amino acids. Still, as long as vegetarians eat a variety of foods with different amino acid profiles, protein isn't an issue. A classic example is combining beans with whole grains.

Like fats, proteins are digested more slowly than carbohydrates (even complex carbs). Therefore they help regulate blood sugar, giving you a steadier supply of energy. Proteins are critical in your diet, but it's important not to overdo it. The Atkins diet and other high-protein diets aren't healthy in the long run. Ideally, protein would make up less than 40 percent of your diet, and you would eat it in combination with fats and complex carbs at every meal or snack. Good sources of protein include free-range eggs, beef, pork, and poultry, as well as seeds, yogurt, and legumes.

🌿 Diane's Story

At age thirty-eight, Diane came to the clinic with symptoms that included fatigue, insomnia, lack of libido, and difficulty concentrating.

She had quit her job as marketing director of a cellular phone company when her second child was born four years earlier. She'd looked forward to spending time with her two small children and exercising more to lose the extra twenty pounds of baby weight she'd gained. But by the time she came in, she barely had the energy to get her daughters to kindergarten and preschool. She dropped them off and returned home to sit on the couch all day, watching television or reading. No matter how much caffeine she drank, she was too tired to exercise or do much during the day. She started to feel better in the late afternoons and got a second wind after dinner—just when her family was getting ready for bed. So after dragging around all day, she had trouble sleeping. She usually tossed and turned until 1 or 2 a.m. and then had trouble getting out of bed at 7 a.m. Her husband was frustrated with her inability to get anything done and didn't understand that her lack of interest in sex had nothing to do with her feelings for him. She just didn't have the energy.

Diane's diet consisted primarily of refined carbohydrates. Dinner was usually pasta or white rice dishes with a few vegetables and just a bit of protein—primarily chicken. She ate virtually no fat, red meat, or fish. She routinely skipped breakfast (as she had for twenty years) and had a salad or leftovers for lunch, snacking on rice cakes and popcorn in the afternoon and drinking several glasses of wine with dinner every night.

Diane wasn't getting enough protein and fat in her diet to balance the refined carbs she was eating. And because refined carbs convert to blood sugar so rapidly, her blood sugar frequently spiked too high for insulin to effectively control. When the body's energy stores are full, glucose is stored as fat, and for Diane (like many of us) this resulted in abdominal weight gain.

Diane's blood tests showed elevated glucose and insulin levels bordering on insulin resistance. Her cortisol was slightly low in the morning, with high levels the rest of the day and at night. Her DHEA was low, indicating that her adrenal glands were starting to tire. Diane's "second wind" in the evenings was actually a disrupted cortisol production pattern: too low in the morning, when it should be high, and then too high when it should be decreasing throughout the day.

The solution was a diet and lifestyle change. Diane's first meeting with the nutritionist was eye-opening. When she realized that eating regularly, particularly first thing in the morning, can prevent the blood sugar and insulin spike that occurs due to eating too much after restricting intake, she started eating a balanced breakfast every morning. She also reduced her intake of refined carbs drastically and substituted vegetables and whole grains. She added protein and fats to her diet at every meal and started supplementing with magnesium, vitamin C, omega-3 fatty acids, maca root, and a good multivitamin every morning. She also took phosphatidylserine and melatonin before bed to help normalize her nighttime cortisol levels.

Once Diane learned that the sugar content in alcohol makes it difficult to stabilize glucose and insulin levels, she cut back her wine consumption to just one glass of wine on weekend nights. She also joined her local gym, met with a personal trainer, and started a weekly yoga class.

At first, Diane felt like she was eating a lot because of the additional fats and protein, but after about a month she noticed that she had more energy in the mornings and was able to cut back on caffeine. Within three months her blood sugar and insulin were in normal ranges and her cortisol levels and production pattern had normalized. By four months Diane's energy level was back to normal and, her husband was delighted to note, so was her interest in sex. She even started to think about looking for a part-time job while her daughters were in school.

ADDITIONAL DIET-RELATED GUIDELINES

There are some basic diet rules that apply to all of us, whether our adrenals are overactive, underactive, or working just fine. Although these guidelines are a good idea for anyone, they're especially beneficial for those whose adrenal health is challenged.

Drink Adequate Water

Our bodies are composed of approximately 70 percent water. Stress can be inherently dehydrating. And when we're under stress, we also tend to drink more coffee, tea, and soda, which are diuretics and increase our need for water. Drink at least 2 quarts (eight 8-ounce glasses) of filtered water every day. To avoid fluoride and chlorine, get a home water filter and filter all the water you use for drinking and cooking. Consider a filter to remove chlorine from bathing water, as well. Keep good water in your car, office, or anywhere you spend a lot of time. Use refillable stainless steel or glass bottles, since plastic leaches unhealthy chemicals into the water over time.

If you have adrenal fatigue and your aldosterone levels are deficient, you should make sure you get enough salt in your diet. Drinking a lot of water without sufficient salt will make your blood levels of sodium lower, and you'll feel worse. Try adding ¼ to 1 teaspoon of salt to a glass of water once or twice a day. To keep your sodium and potassium in balance, be sure to add a potassium-rich food (like bananas) or a potassium supplement when you add salt.

Stay Away from Processed Foods

Try to avoid fast food, canned goods, packaged products, and any other processed food; they're lower in nutrients, and most contain additives that will stress your adrenals. You may feel that you're too busy to cook real meals, but there are plenty of healthful meals that you can put together quickly and easily. Here's an example:

- **Breakfast.** Poach or fry two free-range eggs in a little organic butter over low heat. Fry nitrate-free, organic bacon over low heat; drain on chlorine-free paper towels. Round out the meal with 1 cup of cooked grits or oatmeal, topped with a pat of organic butter and iodized salt.

- **Midmorning snack.** An apple, a banana, or a small bunch of grapes with string cheese.

- **Lunch.** Green salad topped with a piece of broiled wild Alaska salmon. Have some tortilla chips and salsa on the side.

- **Afternoon snack.** A few whole grain crackers topped with cheddar cheese.

🌿 **Dinner.** Broil a free-range chicken breast and cook a cup of brown rice. While you're waiting for these to cook, open a bag of organic prewashed broccoli, steam for five minutes, and dress with olive oil and lemon juice. For dessert, core an apple and fill it with a mixture of 1 teaspoon of brown sugar, chopped pecans or walnuts, chopped raisins, a pat of butter, and ¾ teaspoon of cinnamon. Bake it at 350°F for about forty-five minutes.

🌿 **Evening snack.** Bean soup with a few tortilla chips.

This makes for a wonderfully balanced diet with plenty of high-quality protein, the right fatty acids, and complex carbs in the form of whole grains. You can adjust this basic approach to incorporate whatever meat you'd like and whatever vegetables are in season. Do try to include whole grains, such as quinoa, amaranth, brown rice, barley, buckwheat, bulgur, or millet. You can also eat whole-grain bread and pasta, but always try to have a nonmilled whole grain as well, like brown rice.

Detect and Treat Food Allergies and Sensitivities

Eating foods you're allergic to or sensitive to causes inflammation, which results in the release of cortisol. Excessive or deficient cortisol levels can prevent your body from responding normally to inflammation and result in allergies to foods that never caused problems in the past. Adrenal dysfunction is one of the main reasons so many people develop allergies at midlife. Eliminating foods that cause an inflammatory response removes a huge burden from struggling adrenal glands.

The most common food allergies are to gluten or wheat, eggs, dairy, peanuts, shellfish, tree nuts, soy, and foods in the nightshade family, such as peppers and tomatoes. In addition to exacerbating adrenal fatigue and undermining your immune system, food allergies can damage your stomach lining and hamper your ability to digest food, compromising your ability to get proper nutrition. Studies have found a close connection between gluten sensitivity (celiac disease) and insufficient adrenal function, so be sure to test for food allergies if you have adrenal fatigue (Biagi et al. 2006).

Be Cautious About Eating Soy Products

Eat soy products in moderation, since they can suppress your thyroid function. Soy has been shown to block the conversion of the thyroid hormone T4 to the more active form, T3. Populations that consume lots of soy have a disproportionately high incidence of hypothyroidism. In addition, studies have determined that the plant estrogens in soy can inhibit women's ovaries from producing estrogen and progesterone (Lu et al. 2000). For these reasons, people with hormone deficiencies or imbalances should avoid consuming soy altogether.

Balance Sodium and Potassium

If you consume more salt to support aldosterone production, eat potassium-rich foods to maintain a good balance between sodium and potassium in your body. A potassium to sodium ratio higher than five to one is best. To achieve this, try to get 3 to 4 grams of potassium from potassium-rich foods daily, including meat, fish, nuts, seeds, raisins, figs, dates, bran, bananas, milk, orange juice, cooked beans, avocados, mushrooms, potatoes, apricots, spinach, garlic, yams, and tomatoes.

Restrict Caffeine and Other Stimulants

Caffeine and other stimulants can damage your adrenal function. As much as you may crave stimulants (especially if you have adrenal fatigue), they cause even more stress, forcing your adrenals to try to produce more adrenaline and cortisol, which tires them even further.

Avoid coffee, soft drinks, energy drinks, and energy supplements. Coffee is particularly hard on your adrenals. It triggers increased adrenaline production, while also blocking its removal from your system and intensifying and prolonging its effects. Coffee may allow you to continue working or exercising, but habitual excessive consumption can lead to all of the health problems that excess adrenaline can cause, including looking old before your time. It can also tax fatigued adrenals even further, exacerbating adrenal fatigue.

The situation with tea is not as clear-cut. Studies have found that people who drink black tea had approximately 47 percent lower levels of cortisol in their blood after a stressful event than a control group. Tea didn't appear to reduce the participants' subjective experience of stress, but it did seem to bring stress hormone levels back to normal more quickly (Steptoe et al. 2007).

While you're working to optimize your adrenal function, try to limit beverages with caffeine to one cup a day. If you do consume caffeine, make sure you eat a balanced meal or snack first; this will help stabilize your blood sugar levels throughout the day. As your adrenals heal, you'll find you need stimulants less and can decide on the right amount of caffeine for you.

Avoid Alcohol and Nicotine

Alcohol can damage your adrenals. Though it may seem strange to think of it this way, it's a refined carbohydrate, so it triggers a blood sugar roller coaster and increases insulin production. Since hypoglycemia (an abnormal drop of blood sugar levels) is common in adrenal fatigue, drinking will make it more difficult to balance your blood sugar levels. If you do drink, do so in moderation and try to eat something with your drink, again, to buffer your blood sugar levels.

There is a close tie between adrenal dysfunction and alcoholism (Mendelson, Ogata, and Mello 1971). The body experiences chronic drinking or severe intoxication as a stressor and releases cortisol in response. Yet suddenly stopping chronic drinking is also a form of stress and therefore leads to increased cortisol production (Adinoff et al. 2006). For those with a long-standing drinking habit, patience is key. It will take time to recover adrenal balance.

Alcohol also depletes B vitamins, which are necessary for memory and neurological function, and lowers estrogen levels, which can bring on menopause prematurely.

And while we're on the subject of bad habits, it's also best to avoid smoking or other forms of nicotine. Chronic use results in reduced levels of DHEA (as well as testosterone and progesterone). This reduction in DHEA taxes your adrenals, as they must increase production to compensate.

Slow Down and Eat Mindfully

Moms everywhere say, "Chew your food; don't wolf it down," and they have a good point. Chewing your food thoroughly is critical to proper digestion. Chewing breaks food down into smaller particles and mixes it with enzymes in saliva that begin the process of extracting nutrients. Well-chewed food also has a greater surface area and therefore can be digested more easily. Sufficient saliva in well-chewed food helps relax some of the muscles involved in digestion. Chewing also sends messages to the rest of your gastrointestinal system that promote the digestive process.

Chew your food completely, until it's small enough to be swallowed with ease. The texture should be the same when you swallow whether you're eating steak or bread. To help you slow down, and to make meals a more rewarding experience, savor your food and appreciate its appearance, aromas, textures, and flavors. Also try to eat with friends or family. Socializing as you eat can be pleasant and relaxing, leading to better digestion.

WHERE DOES THIS LEAVE US?

You've tested your levels of key hormones and are treating adrenal hormone deficiencies or excesses by taking vitamins, minerals, other supplements, and bioidentical adrenal hormones as needed. You've adopted a balanced diet—you're on the home stretch!

The last piece of the puzzle of adrenal health is to identify areas in your life that cause chronic stress and learn how to reduce or manage that stress. It's important to identify what habitually triggers your stress response. Remember, stress takes many forms. It may show up in your job, family, other relationships, financial pressures, or in the cumulative weight of all of your responsibilities. Once you identify your stressors, you can work to modify the circumstances, or to modify your response by using healthy coping strategies such as exercising, getting enough sleep, simplifying your life, connecting with others, trying cognitive therapy or mindfulness techniques, being positive and thankful, or praying.

KEY POINTS

- Rather than the traditional three meals a day, eat five or six smaller meals, each containing a combination of protein, complex carbohydrates, and healthy fats. Overall, aim for about 37 percent of calories from protein, 37 percent from carbs, and 26 percent from fat.

- Avoid refined carbohydrates and sugar. Sugar causes vitamin and mineral deficiencies and leads to prolonged high insulin levels, which cause accelerated aging and metabolic damage.

- Eat lots of high-fiber foods. They slow digestion, helping to moderate blood sugar and insulin levels.

- Eat wild fish and meat, dairy products, and eggs from free-range animals for an optimal fatty acid profile: more omega-3s and less omega-6s.

- Don't eat prepared foods marketed as "low-fat." They're typically full of sugar.

- Stay away from trans fats completely—always read ingredients labels.

- Eat organic foods whenever possible.

- Observe the following healthy eating guidelines whenever possible: Drink enough water, avoid processed foods, detect and treat food allergies and sensitivities, use soy products sparingly, balance sodium and potassium, restrict caffeine and other stimulants, avoid alcohol and nicotine, and eat mindfully and chew your food thoroughly.

CHAPTER 8

Managing Stress

Our fight-or-flight response is genetically hardwired to alert us to external threats to our physical survival. This system is highly sensitive and may respond to even small levels of perceived danger. Because of this, our adrenal stress response can be triggered by things we generally believe to be benign, like frustrating personal relationships, day-to-day worries, lack of sleep, or even watching the nightly news. Making some lifestyle changes and incorporating stress management techniques into your daily life can go a long way toward protecting your adrenals.

Stress itself doesn't necessarily have to trigger your fight-or-flight response. It's all in how you perceive and deal with it. You can learn to temper your fight-or-flight response to psychological stressors. Many people believe that challenging situations or people cause their stress, but ultimately it's more about your basic approach to life. If you perceive a potential stressor as a threat, it will trigger the fight-or-flight response and possibly cause you to overreact or become hypervigilant. If, on the other hand, you look at it as a challenge to be met, an opportunity, or simply what is, it's less likely to have a physical effect on your adrenals, allowing you to remain serene and unstressed.

For instance, we all encounter traffic jams now and then. One person sits quietly, listening to an interesting talk show, soothing music, or a book on tape, while another fumes, becoming angrier and angrier. The stressor is the same for both drivers, yet it causes very different physiological responses. This example gets at the heart of the matter: Trying to control the uncontrollable is one of the basic causes of stress. Rather than stressing out, focus on what you can control—your reaction.

When faced with stressful situations that aren't genuine threats, you have a couple of options. You can ignore these stressors. After all, why worry when the situation is beyond your control? Or you can take whatever action is available to you. One thing for sure, getting stressed won't resolve the situation. If you can eliminate the stressor, that's great. If you have no control over the source of stress, you can control how you respond to it.

Recognizing what you can and cannot change is the first step in managing stress. This is why activities like meditation and prayer have proven to be effective in dealing with stress. In both, you strive to give up efforts to control the uncontrollable.

DE-STRESS YOUR LIFE

There are a variety of activities that can help you reduce stress and the resultant wear and tear on your adrenals. We are all unique, and different approaches work for different people, so experiment with a wide range to find those that work best for you. For some people yoga and stretching do the trick, for others a vigorous workout or pursuing a hobby, like gardening or woodwork, is effective, and for yet others prayer or meditation is the answer. Taking a bubble bath, listening to music, reading a good book, or watching a ball game—all can help take your mind off your worries and provide stress relief. It's often the little things that can transform your life and your psychological and physical health.

Identify Your Stressors and How You Respond to Them

Identifying the sources of stress in your life and how you respond to them is the first step in reducing stress. Do you respond to various stressors with a shrug and then move on, or do you often allow them to trigger your flight-or-fight response? It's important to recognize the symptoms and signs of a fight-or-flight reaction; only then can you start to use stress reduction techniques to moderate excessive reactions to events and the excess of stress hormones that results.

We all fall into habits that can increase stress rather than reduce it. We need to regularly reevaluate these behaviors so that we don't add to stress without realizing it. For instance, do you put things off because you feel overwhelmed by how much you have to do? Do you worry about deadlines but then seem to miss them constantly? Procrastination can be the root cause of a great deal of stress. Recognizing and changing this habit can be enormously effective in getting rid of chronic stress due to feeling overwhelmed.

Look closely at your habits and attitudes. Do you tend to blame your stress on other people or events? Until you accept responsibility for your responses, you won't be able to manage them. Next, think about how you currently cope with stress. Do you deal with it in unproductive ways that make it worse, such as drinking, smoking, sleeping or eating too much or too little, using drugs, procrastinating, blaming others, or burying yourself in work, television, or computer activities and withdrawing from family and friends? These strategies may make you feel better in the short term, but they're damaging in the long run. As the old adage says, the definition of insanity is continuing to do the same thing and expecting a different result.

Start a Stress Journal

Sometimes it's hard to identify what's really stressing us. It's human to be oblivious or in denial about everyday stresses and the degree to which they affect us. Keeping a stress journal can help you identify your stressors and how you deal with them. Each time you feel stressed, angry, frustrated, anxious, or scared, record it in your journal, until you start to see patterns emerge. Ideally, you'd record this as soon as possible after the event; alternatively, you could make a journal entry every evening, summing up your day. For each event, note the following:

- **What the stressor is.** Sometimes it's hard to tell, but put down your best guess. For instance, you may feel angry and frustrated and initially blame it on an argument with a coworker. But on further reflection, you might realize that you've heard rumors of layoffs and are feeling powerless about your job and your future.

- **How you feel, both physically and psychologically.** To continue with the example, perhaps you get angry and feel agitated, and your pulse and breathing rate increase.

- **What you do to relieve the stress and make yourself feel better.** Maybe you go to the mall at lunch and buy something for yourself on impulse.

Your journal can help you see the role your behavior plays in feeling stressed. Once you understand it, you can take steps to change the way you respond to stress. In the example above, shopping may make you feel better temporarily, but it doesn't make the most sense if you fear losing your job. As you sort all of this out in your journal, you may realize that a better approach would be to work on your resume and send it out to prospective employers in case you do get laid off. This would be a more productive way to take control and to deal with the stress.

GET REGULAR EXERCISE

Regular physical exercise is a simple and effective way of reducing stress. It provides an outlet for the body when it's in the throes of a fight-or-flight reaction. It's been proven to control cortisol production and help reduce excess adrenaline. It also fosters physical and psychological well-being (Traustadottir, Bosch, and Matt 2005). Exercise also reduces the risk of chronic diseases associated with adrenal dysfunction, such as heart disease, high blood pressure, obesity, osteoporosis, diabetes, and even certain cancers.

An interesting study evaluated men who engaged in regular exercise. They had significantly lower levels of cortisol and heart rate when exposed to a stressor compared with less fit men. They were also much calmer, less anxious, and generally in a better mood (Rimmelea et al. 2007).

Even a short bout of vigorous exercise provides quick stress reduction and counteracts the fight-or-flight response. Any form of activity where you break a sweat for five minutes can effectively help metabolize excess stress hormones. To counteract the negative effects of stress, do jumping jacks or push-ups, run up and down stairs, or do anything that will make you sweat and bring your heart rate up. Frequent, short exercise sessions are easy to fit into almost any schedule. Longer periods of exercise have additional benefits, but for the purpose of stress reduction, short sessions are practical, effective, and beneficial.

For full cardiovascular fitness, try to exercise for thirty to forty-five minutes every other day. Alternate resistance training, like weight lifting, with aerobic exercise, like jogging or cycling. Even walking briskly thirty minutes a day, three times a week helps to reduce cortisol. It also stimulates your lymphatic system, which aids in detoxification and removal of waste products from the body. Swinging your arms while walking pumps lymph fluid through your body. Rebound exercise is also beneficial for the lymphatic system. Jumping on a mini trampoline stimulates lymph flow better than any other form of exercise and also helps build endurance.

A large study of middle-aged women who started walking in their later years showed that walking resulted in a significantly reduced risk of heart disease (Manson et al. 1999). Walking is easy to incorporate into a busy schedule, and walking with a friend is a great way to ensure that you stick to it. When you're tired, the prospect of chatting with a friend while walking is more likely to keep you committed.

The best way to come up with an exercise program that you'll stick with is to find something you enjoy doing that fits with your schedule and lifestyle. However, sometimes it's simply not possible to work regular exercise in to your schedule. Get creative. While standing in line at the grocery store, tense and relax different muscle groups: start with your feet, move to your calves, and so on, moving up through the body.

Don't Overdo It

There is one caution in regard to exercise: In terms of stress reduction, overexercising has the opposite effect—it creates stress rather than moderating it. It causes overproduction of cortisol and can ultimately exhaust your adrenals just like any other chronic stressor. If your exercise program involves sustained cardiovascular exercise, keeping your heart rate over ninety beats per minute, more than three days per week, consider substituting a day or two per week of resistance training or flexibility training, like yoga, to lessen the strain on your adrenals.

Exercising with Adrenal Fatigue

If you have adrenal fatigue, be careful not to overtax yourself at first. Start with mild exercise. If you don't overdo it, regular exercise should help rebuild your adrenals and reduce your fatigue. If you start with an exercise program that's too demanding, it can be difficult to maintain your motivation. It will also heighten your risk of injury or overtaxing your adrenal glands. Consider beginning with slow, peaceful, stretching exercise, such as yoga or tai chi. If your fatigue is severe, you can start with five minutes of stretching exercises once or twice a day. Whatever activity you choose, try to slowly increase the duration and difficulty.

As you start feeling stronger, add some resistance training: any exercise that involves working your muscles against something, like weight training, swimming, or bicycling. The goal is to slowly increase duration and intensity. Remember, overexercising is a form of physical stress and should be avoided at all costs while you're rebuilding your adrenal function.

GET ENOUGH SLEEP AND REST

Stress and the toll it takes on your adrenals can drain you emotionally, mentally, and physically. During times of stress, your body needs help in recovering, and sleep is key. Sleeping helps reduce elevated cortisol levels and restore adrenal function. Yet studies suggest that insomnia can be caused by chronic hyperarousal of the body's stress response system and, unfortunately, sleeplessness causes the body to produce even more cortisol (Vgontzas et al. 1998).

We all know how we feel when we don't get enough sleep: crabby, confused, impatient, intolerant of any stress, and more. Many factors can contribute to sleep problems. First and foremost are hormone imbalances and deficiencies, such as low levels of sex hormones or thyroid hormones, or levels of cortisol that are too low or too high. For optimal sleep, and optimum adrenal health, you need to correct any hormone imbalances.

It's also important to develop good sleep habits. A key strategy is to avoid napping during the day, as it can interfere with nighttime sleep. If you have severe adrenal fatigue, this may seem difficult. As an alternative, try resting with your knees elevated for thirty minutes; this can combat fatigue and help repair your adrenals. Here are a few more tips to help improve your sleep:

- Maintain a consistent sleep schedule. A varying sleep schedule is hard on your body, so try to wake up at the same time every morning, including on weekends.

- Get the right amount of sleep. We all have individual sleep needs; some of us need eight hours, others need more, and others need less.

🖎 Create an optimal sleeping environment. Noise, light, cold, heat, and high or low humidity all can interfere with sleep. Studies show that light decreases the body's production of melatonin, which helps regulate sleep (Bojkowski et al. 1987). Turn off all lights and cover any you can't turn off, such as the LEDs on clocks.

🖎 Exercise regularly. Exercise helps reduce elevated levels of cortisol and adrenaline, which can interfere with sleep.

🖎 Avoid alcohol and caffeine. Both can interfere with sleep. If either disrupts your sleep, cut back on your consumption. Try to avoid caffeine after 2 p.m., and alcohol for several hours before you go to bed.

🖎 Don't take sleeping pills. If you're unable to fall sleep, try supplementing with the body's natural sleep hormone, melatonin, or its precursor, 5-hydroxytryptophan (5-HTP). These are best taken fifteen minutes prior to sleep. As with all hormones, work with your health care practitioner to find your lowest effective dose.

SIMPLIFY YOUR LIFE AND MAKE TIME FOR THE THINGS YOU LOVE

Paring down your responsibilities can make your life much more manageable and take a lot of pressure off your adrenal glands. Cut back on obligations wherever you can. Before you start a new task, add something to your calendar, or put something on your to-do list, ask yourself whether it really needs to be done. You might find that the answer is often no.

Less is also more when it comes to stuff. Clean out your closets, garage, storage unit, or anyplace that excess stuff tends to accumulate. Getting rid of this baggage will streamline your physical and mental space. Be ruthless. Get rid of anything you haven't worn in a year. To ease the pain of getting rid of that $130 jacket you've never worn, offer it to a friend or coworker who's your size. If you don't need something, give it to someone who does. This applies to exercise equipment, electronics, kitchen equipment, furniture, you name it.

Financial worries can be extremely stressful, so try to manage your money in ways that cause the least amount of stress. Implement a thirty-day waiting period before any major purchase. If you still need it after thirty days, think again, then buy it if you absolutely must. You'll probably be surprised by how many things you end up deciding you don't need. Like many impulses, the desire to purchase often subsides after a while. Also take a look at monthly charges for luxuries like satellite radio, extended cable, and so on, and see how many you can eliminate or whittle down.

Part of the simplification process is avoiding procrastination. No matter how trivial they are, to-do items that pile up can cause stress. Be disciplined and don't put off necessary tasks. Do things as they come up—one at a time.

CONNECT WITH OTHERS

Social and emotional support is very effective in helping us handle stress. A strong sense of community, whether it's with your neighborhood, your church, the company you work for, a book club, or some other group, is important. It will help you feel connected and supported, especially in tough times.

Emotional support from family and friends is a buffer against extremes of emotion that can cause swings of cortisol and adrenaline production. Recent studies show that just hearing your mother's voice can significantly reduce cortisol levels (Seltzer, Ziegler, and Pollak 2010). Another study demonstrated that friendship can reduce our perception of how stressful obstacles are. Researchers had participants stand at the base of a steep hill and asked them to estimate how hard it would be to climb. Those accompanied by a friend thought the hill was less steep than those who were alone (Schnall et al. 2008). And when participants were alone, if they just thought of a supportive friend they saw the hill as less steep. In addition, the longer participants had known their friends, the more manageable they estimated the hill to be.

Research has also uncovered links between health and friendship. In a study at Harvard, researchers found that breast cancer patients without a network of friends were four times more likely to die from the disease than those with ten or more close friends (Kroenke et al. 2006).

Women often find it easier to connect with other people than men do, but everyone needs someone to decompress with. Whether you get together for shopping, a ball game, or just over the phone, spending time with friends has been shown to reduce stress and give us a sense of belonging, security, and increased self-worth (Kikusui, Winslow, and Mori 2006).

Identify Stressful Relationships

While personal relationships can be lifesavers, they can also be a source of ongoing stress and the catalyst for adrenal hormone production. Whenever possible, avoid people who stress you out, or find a way to respond to them differently. If a friend, family member, or significant other consistently causes stress in your life, it's affecting your adrenals and you need to make a change. You have several options: You can mend the relationship, end it, limit the amount of time you spend with that person, or work on how you respond to them.

One easy way to reduce stress in a relationship is to stay away from hot-button topics. If you get upset over a particular topic like religion or politics, politely refuse to discuss it. If you find yourself repeatedly arguing about the same thing, stop the madness and change the subject. If this doesn't work, excuse yourself from the discussion.

Define boundaries or limits on how other people interact with you. Decide what you will and won't tolerate in your life. Then communicate this firmly, consistently, and pleasantly to people who try to cross those boundaries. When others are doing something that makes you begin to feel resentful, angry, or frustrated, let them know immediately. If you don't, chances are the situation will escalate, heightening your stress response.

One caveat with this approach: It would also be a good idea to examine your responses to see whether you might be overreacting. Take a moment to take a few deep breaths and look at the situation objectively before calling the other person on their behavior. And keep in mind that other people generally fall in the category of things we cannot change.

Take A Relationship Inventory

It's important to determine if you have toxic people in your life: people who make you feel uncomfortable, anxious, sad, or bad about yourself, or who bring on any other negative emotions. Look at your friends, family, children, spouse or significant other, and coworkers to see whether any of them could be adding to your stress.

First think of the positives: What does this person add to your life? Next, consider the negatives: How do you feel after you've been with the person? How do the person's actions affect you? If you tend to feel angry, frustrated, or tired when you're with certain people, chances are the relationship is setting off your stress response and you need to make changes.

Finally, weigh the positives against the negatives. If the negatives outweigh the positives, write down your thoughts about boundaries you need to set or changes you need to make in order to reduce stress.

Potential Stressor	Positive	Negative	Thoughts
Example: Parents	*Mother: She's always there for me.*	*She wants me to visit her every day.*	*Tell her I can't visit daily right now. I'll plan on being there Sunday and Wednesday evenings for the time being.*
Parents			
Siblings			
Spouse or significant other			

Children			
Friends			
Coworkers			
Other			
Other			
Other			

You have several choices in deciding what to do about any negative relationships you've identified. You can try to mend the relationship, but if you've tried to mend a relationship and nothing is working, it's probably time to move on. If you decide to end a relationship, realize that this too can be stressful. If the person isn't a part of your daily life, you can just let the relationship fade. Don't call or return calls, and eventually you'll probably lose touch without too much pain or drama.

When you don't want to end a relationship but it's causing you more stress than you need, accepting that you can't change other people is the first step. Instead, focus on what you can change: yourself and your reactions. You might try to develop more acceptance of things that annoy you, or you might choose to not participate in the types of interactions that stress you. If there's mutual love, caring, and respect and you're willing to compromise, you can end up with a stronger, healthier relationship.

You may also find that you're stressed more by the cumulative weight of your relationships than by any particular relationship. Perhaps you're run ragged by family responsibilities. Maybe you have kids at home to take care of, as well as parents down the street who are aging and need help. If there are just too many people tugging at you, you need to find a way for others to take up some of the slack and free you from some of the burden.

TRY COGNITIVE THERAPY

Cognitive therapy is a field of psychology focused on changing dysfunctional thinking, behavior, and emotional responses—all of which can be stressors in their own right. Cognitive therapy helps people develop skills to identify and modify thoughts that are distorted and counterproductive.

For example, it's common to dwell on past mistakes. Distorted thinking can cause us to extrapolate that we can't do anything right, starting a downward spiral that leads to imagining that everything we do is wrong and that we'll never amount to anything. This negative programming colors everything, making us less willing to take chances and fostering a belief that bad things are going to happen. Unfortunately, this often becomes a self-fulfilling prophecy. If we feel categorically bad about ourselves, we may be disinclined to even try to accomplish things that are important to us, fueling the cycle.

Cognitive therapy can be helpful in changing negative thought patterns and dysfunctional behaviors. It can help us look at our situation and circumstances in a more accepting and positive light. With time, stressors will seem less threatening and less likely to trigger the stress response.

PRACTICE MINDFULNESS TECHNIQUES

Mindfulness-based relaxation techniques can be very effective in reducing stress and cortisol levels. There are many to choose from, including meditation, progressive relaxation, deep breathing, and visualization. Exercises such as yoga and tai chi combine mindfulness and breathing with physical exercise. The goal of these techniques is to quiet the mind and detach from the endless stream of thoughts constantly surging through our minds. There's a tendency for this stream of thoughts to dwell on the negative, such as worries and fears, so not only does it distract us, it can also trigger the fight-or-flight response.

Although meditation originated in religious and spiritual traditions, it isn't an inherently religious practice. People of all faiths can practice and benefit from meditation. Meditation can be anything from simply sitting quietly for a few minutes to guided imagery and visualization to more complex practices, but in general meditation involves becoming mindful of your thoughts, feelings, and sensations in a nonjudgmental way. With time and practice, you can learn to observe emotions and thoughts without responding to them.

Meditation will also train you to pay attention to your response to stressful events and even help you modulate your body's response. Clinical studies have proven that meditation relieves stress and reduces cortisol levels (MacLean et al. 1997).

Deep breathing for a few minutes a day can have effects similar to meditation and help modify the messages that your body sends to your brain, reducing cortisol and adrenaline production. Try breathing in through your nose for a count of six. Then hold your breath for a count of six, and then breath out for a count of six. This is a good way to de-stress in the middle of a hectic day or in a stressful situation. Try it the next time something sets you off and you feel your heart racing. You may be amazed at how quickly and effectively it moderates your response.

BE POSITIVE AND THANKFUL

Cultivating a positive attitude is critical to adrenal health and stress relief. Believing that good things will happen to you, rather than bad, can reduce stress (Scheier and Carver 1993). Put life in perspective. Your situation could always be worse than it is. Focus on the positives instead of the negatives. Admittedly, sometimes this is hard. The media constantly presents a negative view of the world. To maintain equanimity, it's important to distance yourself from things you can't affect. In fact, most psychologists recommend taking a periodic holiday from news to maintain mental health and balance.

Laughter is an even better solution to stress, so try to see the humor in life. Your body's response to laughter is similar to its response to moderate exercise; it can lower cortisol and adrenaline levels (Berk, Tan, and Berk 2008; Berk et al. 1988).

Although it can be hard to see while you're in the midst of them, most negative situations also contain positives. Approaching life with an attitude of thankfulness takes the focus away from the negative and puts it on the positive. Do you know people who are able to maintain a relatively positive attitude regardless of what's happening around them? These people are generally able to see blessings in the middle of adversity and are grateful for what they do have. Being grateful makes us more receptive: When we expect good things to happen, they often do. And at a minimum, we'll be more likely to notice the good things that are indeed so often happening all around us.

Add a Gratitude Section to Your Stress Journal

Gratitude can be learned. It may come more easily to some of us than others, but making a point of acknowledging what you can be thankful for will help make it a regular part of your life. Take a minute now to think about what you're grateful for. Then, make a list below of people, things, and events for which you're grateful. These could be anything from your pet, your house, or your spouse to your upcoming vacation or getting a perfect haircut.

_____

_____

_____

_____

_____

_____

_____

_____

Next, add a daily gratitude section to your stress journal. After you write about what stressors you encountered each day, list things that you're grateful for. Don't censor your entries. If you're grateful that you found the perfect rug for your entryway, write it down. If you saved hundreds of dollars on your insurance renewal, be grateful for it. Nothing is too small or insignificant to write down. As you start to see all of these good things mount up, it will be easier to count your blessings. If you do hit a bump in the road, reading back through the gratitude entries in your journal will help put things in perspective.

Review these entries once a week. You'll probably find that it gets much easier to find things that you're grateful for when you're attuned to looking for them. As your list grows, so will your positive outlook.

PRAY AND LET GO

Much of our daily stress comes from trying to control and change things. Prayer acknowledges that some higher power is in charge, not us. By letting go of those things in your life that you can't control, you relieve yourself of a huge burden. You also allow others to be responsible for themselves. Prayer has been proven to reduce stress and even normalize cortisol levels. In one study among women with fibromyalgia, those with strong or moderately strong religious beliefs had a more typical cortisol production pattern, with high levels in the morning and low levels in the evening. In comparison, those with less strong religious beliefs had a relatively flattened cortisol rhythms (Dedert et al. 2004).

Letting go of the need to try to control everything and turning your troubles over to a higher power is the basis of successful addiction programs such as Alcoholics Anonymous and other 12-step programs. The Serenity Prayer, written by Reinhold Niebuhr in 1943 and used in many of these programs, articulates our need for strength and peace when we're in the midst of uncertainty, turmoil, or despair: "God, grant me the serenity to accept the things I cannot change; courage to change the things I can; and wisdom to know the difference."

Changing the things we can gives us a sense of control over our environment. If you're feeling stressed, take charge. Get more exercise, schedule activities with friends, make positive changes to relationships that are adding to your stress, clean out closets, meditate, or practice other stress reduction techniques—all can contribute to positive changes. Plus, focusing on the things we can change keeps our minds off the things we can't.

Along with prayer goes forgiveness—for ourselves and for others. When we make mistakes we need to be gentle and forgiving with ourselves. The damage is already done; learn from it and move on. Not only is excessive guilt unproductive, it's been shown to result in higher levels of cortisol and DHEA—as much as 23 percent higher in one study (McCraty et al. 1998).

And when others harm us, we also need to forgive them and put it behind us. Holding on to resentments is one of the easiest ways to perpetuate stress. It starts to color the way we look at the world and makes us expect the worst from others. Forgiving someone doesn't mean you exonerate them from responsibility or that what happened is okay. It's an act of letting go, freeing ourselves from anger, pain, and resentment. There's an old saying that sums it up: Lack of forgiveness is like drinking poison and hoping the other guy dies. Holding on to resentment creates ongoing stress and compounds the original insult or hurt.

WHERE DOES THIS LEAVE US?

The key to maximizing adrenal health is managing stress by taking charge of your emotions, thoughts, and schedule and the way you deal with problems. Taking charge allows you to balance your life, leaving time for work, relationships, and relaxation, and time to pursue your passions.

Start today! You can't go wrong with any approach that will help you enjoy life more, reduce stress, and heal your adrenals.

KEY POINTS

- Many people believe that situations or people cause their stress, but we can affect how we respond to stress by adopting an optimistic approach to life. Expect good things to happen, not bad.

- In order to resolve stress, it's important to evaluate what part you play in creating it. Think about what caused your stress, how you feel and respond when you get stressed, and what you do to relieve stress and make yourself feel better.

- Avoid people who stress you out. Mend or end toxic relationships, or limit the amount of time you spend with these people. Alternatively, you may need to work on your own responses to develop more tolerance for and acceptance of others.

- Proven stress-reduction techniques include exercising, getting enough sleep, simplifying your life, connecting with others, trying cognitive therapy, meditating, being positive and thankful, and praying

Conclusion

I hope I've persuaded you to take your adrenal health seriously. I learned the hard way how important the adrenal glands are to overall health, but there's no need for you to suffer the same fate. If anything you've read in this book makes you suspect that your adrenal glands are under-producing or overproducing hormones, call your doctor or find a doctor who specializes in adrenal health so you can get started on the process of evaluating and optimizing your adrenal function.

My goal has been to help you understand your symptoms and what they mean, and generally make sense out of your personal situation. You need to be able to read the symptoms and signs that tell you that your stress response has been triggered: racing heartbeat, shallow breathing, deep sighing, muscle tension, upset stomach, headache, and so on. You also need to be alert to signs that you're suffering from a long-term or chronic stress response, such as depression, anxiety, hopeless-ness, fear, or problems with concentration or memory.

Resolving these symptoms may be as easy as treating chronic infections, changing your diet, or using stress management techniques like meditation, acupuncture, or thinking positively and enjoying life more. Using these and the other tools you've learned in this book, you can success-fully manage your own health. Be confident that you will experience renewed vitality, energy, and joy, and that you don't have to suffer the ill health that adrenal dysfunction can cause. Through methodical and wise application of everything you've learned here, and with the collaboration of a good doctor, you have everything you need to regain or maintain good health.

I know I've given you a lot of information to consider and digest. Some of it may seem daunting at first, but don't despair. Go back to the chapters and sections that apply to you and reread them a few times. It will all start to make sense. Don't let the situation overwhelm you; just take it one step at a time. And always remember, your health and well-being are well worth the investment of your time and energy.

I wish you the courage of your new convictions. Good luck in your quest, and let me know how you do.

In health,

Kathy Simpson

ksimpson@hormoneresource.com

Resources

The following are resources for locating physicians who may specialize in adrenal testing and treatment. The first six include physician locator options on their websites. You simply enter your zip code or city and the website lists any doctors in your area.

American College for Advancement in Medicine (ACAM)
(800) 532-3688
www.acamnet.org

American Academy of Anti-Aging Medicine (A4M)
(888) 997-0112
www.worldhealth.net

American Holistic Medical Association
(216) 292-6644
www.holisticmedicine.org

American Association of Naturopathic Physicians

(866) 538-2267

www.naturopathic.org

This organization is relevant to California and other states where naturopaths can prescribe bio-identical hormones. Check to see if naturopaths are licensed to prescribe drugs in your particular state.

Health Professionals Directory

www.healthprofs.com

Thyroid Doctors

www.thyroid-info.com

International Academy of Compounding Pharmacists (IACP)

(800) 927-4227

www.iacprx.org.

Compounding pharmacies make individualized bioidentical hormones, and staff members generally know which local doctors prescribe them.

Phone Book

Look in the yellow pages under "physicians." Hormone specialists often advertise themselves as holistic physicians.

References

Abou-Raya, A., and S. Abou-Raya. 2006. Inflammation: A pivotal link between autoimmune diseases and atherosclerosis. *Autoimmunity Reviews* 5(5):331-337.

Adinoff, B., K. Ruether, S. Krebaum, A. Iranmanesh, and M. J. Williams. 2006. Increased salivary cortisol concentrations during chronic alcohol intoxication in a naturalistic clinical sample of men. *Alcoholism: Clinical and Experimental Research* 27(9):1420-1427.

Akwa, Y., and E. E. Baulieu. 1999. Neurosteroids: Behavioural aspects and physiological implications. *Journal de la Société de Biologie* 103(30):293-298.

Al-Dujaili, E., R. Chalmers, and M. Sharp. 2007. Does ginseng ingestion influence salivary testosterone and DHEA levels in females. *Endocrine Abstracts* 13:285.

Alevritis, E., F. Sarubbi, R. Jordan, and A. N. Peiris. 2003. Infectious causes of adrenal insufficiency. *Southern Medical Journal* 96(9):888-890.

Alexander, R. W. 1994. Inflammation and coronary artery disease. *New England Journal of Medicine* 33(7):468-469.

American Heart Association. 1961. Dietary fat and its relation to heart attacks and strokes. *Journal of the American Medical Association* 175:389-391.

Armas, L. G., B. W. Hollis, and R. P. Heaney. 2004. Vitamin D_2 is much less effective than vitamin D_3 in humans. *Journal of Clinical Endocrinology and Metabolism* 89(11):5387-5391.

Arnsten, A., and P. Goldman-Rakic. 1998. Noise stress impairs prefrontal cortical cognitive function in monkeys: Evidence for a hyperdopaminergic mechanism. *Archives of General Psychiatry* 55(4):362-368.

Barr, R., T. Kurth, M. J. Stampfer, J. E. Buring, C. H. Hennekens, and J. M. Gaziano. 2007. Aspirin and decreased adult-onset asthma: Randomized comparisons from the Physicians' Health Study. *American Journal of Respiratory and Critical Care Medicine* 175(2):120-125.

Benvenga, S., A. Toscano, C. Rodolico, G. Vita, and F. Trimarchi. 2001. Endocrine evaluation for muscle pain. *Journal of the Royal Society of Medicine* 94(8):405-407.

Bergendahl, M., M. L. Vance, A. Iranmanesh, M. O. Thorner, and J. D. Veldhuis. 1996. Fasting as a metabolic stress paradigm selectively amplifies cortisol secretory burst mass and delays the time of maximal nyctohemeral cortisol concentrations in healthy men. *Journal of Clinical Endocrinology and Metabolism* 81(2):692-699.

Berk, L. S., S. A. Tan, and D. Berk. 2008. Cortisol and catecholamine stress hormone decrease is associated with the behavior of perceptual anticipation of mirthful laughter. *The FASEB Journal* 22:946.11.

Berk, L. S., S. A. Tan, S. Nehlsen-Cannarella, et al. 1988. Humor associated laughter decreases cortisol and increases spontaneous lymphocyte blastogenesis. *Clinical Research* 36(3):435A.

Biagi, F., J. Campanella, A. Soriani, A. Vailati, and G. R. Corazza. 2006. Prevalence of coeliac disease in Italian patients affected by Addison's disease. *Scandinavian Journal of Gastroenterology* 41(3):302-305.

Bijlsma, J. W. J, R. H. Straub, A. T. Masi, R. G. Lahita, and M. Cutolo. 2002. Neuroendocrine immune mechanisms in rheumatic diseases. *Trends in Immunology* 23(2):59-61.

Bojkowski, C. J., M. E. Aldhous, J. English, et al. 1987. Suppression of nocturnal plasma melatonin and 6-sulphatoxymelatonin by bright and dim light in man. *Hormone and Metabolic Research* 19(9):437-440.

Bornstein, S., C. Stratakis, and G. Chrousos. 1999. Adrenocortical tumors: Recent advances in basic concepts and clinical management. *Annals of Internal Medicine* 130(9):759-771.

Boscarino, J. A. 2004. Posttraumatic stress disorder and physical illness: Results from clinical and epidemiologic studies. *Annals of the New York Academy of Sciences* 1032:141-153.

Brody, S., R. Preut, K. Schommer, and T. H. Schürmeyer. 2002. A randomized controlled trial of high dose ascorbic acid for reduction of blood pressure, cortisol, and subjective responses to psychological stress. *Psychopharmacology* 159(3):319-324.

Brot, C., P. Vestergaard, N. Kolthoff, J. Gram, A. P. Hermann, and O. H. Sùrensen. 2001. Vitamin D status and its adequacy in healthy Danish perimenopausal women: Relationships to dietary intake, sun exposure, and serum parathyroid hormone. *British Journal of Nutrition* (86)1:S97-S103.

Brown, E., E. Varghese, and B. McEwen. 2004. Association of depression with medical illness: Does cortisol play a role? *Biological Psychiatry* (55)1:1-9.

Bunevicius, R., G. Kazanavicius, R. Zalinkevicius, and A. J. Prange. 1999. Effects of thyroxine as compared with thyroxine plus triiodothyronine in patients with hypothyroidism. *New England Journal of Medicine* 340(6):424-429.

Burke, H. M., M. C. Davis, C. Otte, and D. C. Mohr. 2005. Depression and cortisol responses to psychological stress: A meta-analysis. *Psychoneuroendocrinology* 30(9):846-856.

Burton, J. M., S. Kimball, R. Vieth, et al. 2010. A phase I/II dose-escalation trial of vitamin D3 and calcium in multiple sclerosis. *Neurology* 74(23):1852-1859.

Catena, C., G. Colussi, E. Nadalini, et al. 2008. Cardiovascular outcomes in patients with primary aldosteronism after treatment. *Archives of Internal Medicine* 168(1):80-85.

Chae, C. U., R. T. Lee, N. Rifai, and P. M. Ridker. 2001. Blood pressure and inflammation in apparently healthy men. *Hypertension* 38(3):399-403.

Chiodini, I., G. Adda, E. P. Beck-Peccoz, E. Orsi, B. Ambrosi, and M. Arosio. 2007. Cortisol secretion in patients with type 2 diabetes: Relationship with chronic complications [author reply]. *Diabetes Care* 30:e50.

Chiodini, I., M. Toriontano, V. Carnevale, V. Trischitta, and A. Scillitani. 2008. Skeletal involvement in adult patients with endogenous hypercortisolism. *Journal of Endocrinological Investigation* 31(3):267-276.

Chrousos, G. P., D. Detera-Wadleigh, and M. Karl. 1993. Syndromes of glucocorticoid resistance. *Annals of Internal Medicine* 119(11):1113-1124.

Chrousos, G. P., D. Torpy, and P. Gold. 1998. Interactions between the hypothalamic-pituitary-adrenal axis and the female reproductive system: Clinical implications. *Annals of Internal Medicine* 129(3):229-240.

Cutolo, M., A. Sulli, and C. Pizzorni, et al. 2002. Cortisol, dehydroepiandrosterone sulfate, and androstenedione levels in patients with polymyalgia rheumatica during twelve months of glucocorticoid therapy. *Annals of the New York Academy of Sciences* 966:91-96.

Deaton, M. A., J. E. Glorioso, and D. B. McLean. 1999. Congenital adrenal hyperplasia: Not really a zebra. *American Family Physician* 59(5):1190-1196.

Dedert, E., J. L. Studts, I. Weissbecker, P. G. Salmon, P. L. Banis, and S. E. Sephton. 2004. Religiosity may help preserve the cortisol rhythm in women with stress-related illness. *International Journal of Psychiatry in Medicine* 34(1):61-77.

Delarue, J., O. Matzinger, C. Binnert, P. Schneiter, P. Chioléro, and L. Tappy. 2003. Fish oil prevents the adrenal activation elicited by mental stress in healthy men. *Diabetes Metabolism* 29(3):289-295.

Demeneix, B. A., and N. E. Henderson. 1978. Thyroxine metabolism in active and torpid ground squirrels, *Spermophilus richardsoni*. *General and Comparative Endocrinology* 35(1):86-92.

Dinan, T., E. Quigley, S. Ahmed, et al. 2006. Hypothalamic-pituitary-gut axis dysregulation in irritable bowel syndrome: Plasma cytokines as a potential biomarker. *Gastroenterology* 130(2):304-311.

Durrant-Peatfield, B. 2003. *Your Thyroid and How to Keep It Healthy*. London: Hammersmith Press.

Epel, E. S., B. McEwen, T. Seeman, et al. 2000. Stress and body shape: Stress-induced cortisol secretion is consistently greater among women with central fat. *Psychosomatic Medicine* 62(5):623-632.

Feng, J. T., and C. P. Hu. 2005. Dysfunction of releasing adrenaline in asthma by nerve growth factor. *Medical Hypotheses* 65(6):1043-1046.

Ferrari, E., L. Cravello, B. Muzzoni, et al. 2001. Age-related changes of the hypothalamic-pituitary-adrenal axis: Pathophysiological correlates. *European Journal of Endocrinology* 144(4):319-329.

Field, T., M. Hernandez-Reif, M. Diego, S. Schanberg, and C. Kuhn. 2005. Cortisol decreases and serotonin and dopamine increase following massage therapy. *International Journal of Neuroscience* 115(10):1397-1413.

Frank, A. J., L. Scheer, and R. M. Buijs. 1999. Light affects morning salivary cortisol in humans. *Journal of Clinical Endocrinology and Metabolism* 84(9):3395-3398.

Frost, G., A. Leeds, C. Doré, S. Madeiros, S. Brading, and A. Dornhorst. 1999. Glycaemic index as a determinant of serum HDL-cholesterol concentration. *Lancet* 353(9158):1045-1048.

Gadsby, P. 2004. The Inuit paradox: How can people who gorge on fat and rarely see a vegetable be healthier than we are? *Discover Magazine* 25(10).

Galisteo, M., J. Duarte, and A. Zarzuelo. 2008. Effects of dietary fibers on disturbances clustered in the metabolic syndrome. *Journal of Nutritional Biochemistry* 19(2):71-84.

García-Borreguero, D., T. A. Wehr, O. Larrosa, et al. 2000. Glucocorticoid replacement is permissive for rapid eye movement sleep and sleep consolidation in patients with adrenal insufficiency. *Journal of Clinical Endocrinology and Metabolism* (85)11:4201-4206.

Gell, J. S., J. Oh, W. E. Rainey, and B. R. Carr. 1998. Effect of estradiol on DHEAS production in the human adrenocortical cell line, H295R. *Journal of the Society for Gynecologic Investigation* 5(3):144-148.

George, R., and R. Bhopal. 1995. Fat composition of free living and farmed sea species: Implications for human diet and sea-farming techniques. *British Food Journal* 97(8):19-22.

Golf, S. W., O. Happel, V. Graef, and K. E. Seim. 1984. Plasma aldosterone, cortisol, and electrolyte concentrations in physical exercise after magnesium supplementation. *Journal of Clinical Chemistry and Clinical Biochemistry* 22(11):717-721.

Gordon, G. G., and A. L. Southren. 1977. Thyroid hormone effects on steroid hormone metabolism. *Bulletin of the New York Academy of Medicine* 53(3):241-259.

Gorham, E. D., C. F. Garland, F. C. Garland, et al. 2007. Optimal vitamin D status for colorectal cancer prevention: A quantitative meta analysis. *American Journal of Preventative Medicine* 32(3):210-216.

Gotoh, S., N. Nishimura, O. Takahashi, et al. 2008. Adrenal function in patients with community-acquired pneumonia. *European Respiratory Journal* 31(6):1268-1273.

Grootveld, M., C. Silwood, P. Claxson, B. Serra, and M. Viana. 2001. Health effects of oxidized heated oils. *Foodservice Research International* 13(1):41-55.

Guth, L., Z. Zhang, and E. Roberts. 1994. Key role for pregnenolone in combination therapy that promotes recovery after spinal cord injury. *Proceedings of the National Academy of Sciences* 91(25):12308-12312.

Haye, B., J. L. Aublin, S. Champion, B. Lambert, and C. Jacquemin. 1985. Chronic and acute effects of forskolin on isolated thyroid cell metabolism. *Molecular Cell Endocrinology* 43(1):41-50.

Heim, C., and C. B. Nemeroff. 2001. The role of childhood trauma in the neurobiology of mood and anxiety disorders: Preclinical and clinical studies. *Biological Psychiatry* 49(12):1023-1039.

Hellhammer, J., E. Fries, C. Buss, et al. 2004. Effects of soy lecithin phosphatidic acid and phosphatidylserine complex (PAS) on the endocrine and psychological responses to mental stress. *Stress* 7(2):119-126.

Hertoghe, T. 2006. *The Hormone Handbook.* Surrey, UK: International Medical Publications.

Hickling, P., R. K. Jacoby, and J. R. Kirwan. 1998. Joint destruction after glucocorticoids are withdrawn in early rheumatoid arthritis. *British Journal of Rheumatology* 37(9):930-936.

Hinson, J. P., and P. W. Raven. 1999. DHEA deficiency syndrome: A new term for old age? *Journal of Endocrinology* 163(1):1-5.

Hoffman, L. C. 2006. Game and venison: Meat for the modern consumer. *Meat Science* 74(1):197-208.

Hollifield, M., N. Sinclair-Lian, T. D. Warner, and R. Hammerschlag. 2007. Acupuncture for posttraumatic stress disorder: A randomized controlled pilot trial. *Journal of Nervous and Mental Disease* 195(6):504-513.

Honk, J., D. Schutter, E. Hermans, and P. Putnam. 2003. Low cortisol levels and the balance between punishment sensitivity and reward dependency. *Neuroendocrinology* (14)15:1993-1996.

Jefferies, W. M. 2004. *Safe Uses of Cortisol*. Springfield, IL: C. C. Thomas.

Jenkins, D., T. M. Wolever, R. H. Taylor, H. M. Barker, and H. Fielden. 1980. Exceptionally low blood glucose response to dried beans: Comparison with other carbohydrate foods. *British Medical Journal* 281:578-580.

Jezova, D., R. Duncko, M. Lassanova, M. Kriska, and F. Moncek. 2002. Reduction of rise in blood pressure and cortisol release during stress by *Ginkgo biloba* extract (EGb 761) in healthy volunteers. *Journal of Physiology and Pharmacology* 53(3):337-348.

Jiang, S., J. Lee, Z. Zhang, P. Inserra, D. Solkoff, and R. R. Watson. 1998. Dehydroepiandrosterone synergizes with antioxidant supplements for immune restoration in old as well as retrovirus-infected mice. *Journal of Nutritional Biochemistry* 9(7):362-369.

Johnson, R., L. J. Appel, M. Brands, et al. 2009. Dietary sugars intake and cardiovascular health. *Circulation* 120(11):1101-1020.

Johnson, R., and T. Gower. 2009. *The Sugar Fix: The High-Fructose Fallout That Is Making You Sick and Fat*. New York: Rodale.

Kalman, D., S. Feldman, R. Feldman, H. Schwartz, D. Krieger, and R. Garrison. 2008. Effect of a proprietary *Magnolia* and *Phellodendron* extract on stress levels in healthy women: A pilot, double-blind, placebo-controlled clinical trial. *Nutrition Journal* 7:11.

Kalmijn, S., L. Launer, R. Stolk, et al. 1998. A prospective study on cortisol, dehydroepiandrosterone sulfate, and cognitive function in the elderly. *Journal of Clinical Endocrinology and Metabolism* 83(10):3487-3492.

Kariyawasam, S., F. Zaw, and S. Handley. 2002. Reduced salivary cortisol in children with comorbid attention deficit hyperactivity disorder and oppositional defiant disorder. *Neuroendocrinology Letters* 23(1):45-48.

Katz, F., P. Romfh, J. A. Smith, E. Roper, and J. Barnes. 1975. Combination contraceptive effects on monthly cycle of plasma aldosterone, renin activity, and renin substrate. *Acta Endocrinologica* 79(2):295-300.

Keith, K., H. Nicholson, and S. Assinder. 2006. Effect of increasing ratio of estrogen:androgen on proliferation of normal human prostate stromal and epithelial cells, and the malignant cell line LNCaP. *Prostate* 66(1):105-114.

Kelly, G. 2001. *Rhodiola rosea*: A possible plant adaptogen. *Alternative Medicine Review* 6(3):293-302.

Kikusui, T., J. Winslow, and Y. Mori. 2006. Social buffering: Relief from stress and anxiety. *Philosophical Transactions of the Royal Society B: Biological Sciences* 361(1476):2215-2228.

Kirschbaum, C., J. Prüssner, A. Stone, et al. 1995. Persistent high cortisol responses to repeated psychological stress in a subpopulation of healthy men. *Psychosomatic Medicine* 57(5):468-474.

Kish, S. J., K. Shannak, and O. Hornykiewicz. 1988. Uneven patterns of dopamine loss in the striatum of patients with idiopathic Parkinson's disease: Pathophysiologic and clinical implication. *New England Journal of Medicine* 318(14):876-880.

Klaitman, V., and Y. Almog. 2003. Corticosteroids in sepsis: A new concept for an old drug. *Israel Medical Association Journal* 5(1):51-54.

Kroenke, C. H., L. D. Kubzansky, E. S. Schernhammer, M. D. Holmes, and I. Kawachi. 2006. Social networks, social support, and survival after breast cancer diagnosis. *Journal of Clinical Oncology* 24(7):1105-1111.

Kumari, M., E. Badrick, J. Ferrie, A. Perski, M. Marmot, and T. Chandola. 2009. Self-reported sleep duration and sleep disturbance are independently associated with cortisol secretion in the Whitehall II Study. *Journal of Clinical Endocrinology and Metabolism* 94(12):4801-4809.

Laughlin, G., and E. Barret-Connor. 2000. Sexual dimorphism in the influence of advanced aging on adrenal hormone levels: The Rancho Bernardo Study. *Journal of Clinical Endocrinology* 85(10):3561-3568.

Lazarus, R., and S. Folkman. 1984. *Stress, Appraisal, and Coping.* New York: Springer-Verlag.

Lee, A. L., W. O. Ogle, and R. M. Sapolsky. 2002. Stress and depression: Possible links to neuron death in the hippocampus. *Bipolar Disorders* 4(2):117-128.

Lee, S., S. Yin, M. Lee, W. Tsai, and C. Sim. 1982. Effects of acupuncture on serum cortisol level and dopamine beta-hydroxylase activity in normal Chinese. *American Journal of Chinese Medicine* 10(1-4):62-69.

Li, Z. R., M. H. Shen, and Y. J. Peng. 2005. Progress in researches on the effect of acupuncture in antagonizing oxygen stress. *Chinese Journal of Integrative Medicine* 11(2):156-160.

Liu, J., and A. Mori. 1999. Stress, aging, and brain oxidative damage. *Neurochemical Research* 24(11):1479-1497.

Loesche, W. J. 1994. Periodontal disease as a risk factor for heart disease. *Compendium* 15(8):976, 978-982, 985-986.

Lu, L., K. Anderson, J. Grady, F. Kohen, and M. Nagamani. 2000. Decreased ovarian hormones during a soya diet: Implications for breast cancer prevention. *Cancer Research* 60(15):4112-4121.

MacLean, C., K. Walton, S. Wenneberg, et al. 1997. Effects of the Transcendental Meditation program on adaptive mechanisms: Changes in hormone levels and responses to stress after 4 months of practice. *Psychoneuroendocrinology* 22(4):277-295.

Manson, J. E., F. B. Hu, J. W. Rich-Edwards, et al. 1999. A prospective study of walking as compared with vigorous exercise in the prevention of coronary heart disease in women. *New England Journal of Medicine* 341(9):650-658.

Mariani, E., G. Ravaglia, P. Forti, et al. 1999. Vitamin D, thyroid hormones, and muscle mass influence natural killer (NK) innate immunity in healthy nonagenarians and centenarians. *Clinical and Experimental Immunology* 116(1):19-27.

Martorell, P. M., B. O. Roep, and J. W. Smit. 2002. Autoimmunity in Addison's disease. *Netherlands Journal of Medicine* 60(7):269-275.

Masi, A., R. Chatterton, T. Fecht, et al. 1998. Dissociation of serum dehydroepiandrosterone sulfate (DHEAS) and cortisol levels in younger premenopausal women prior to onset of rheumatoid arthritis (RA) before age 50: Results of a prospective, controlled study. *Arthritis and Rheumatism* 41:559.

Mason, Z. 2010. The Scientist: Thomas Overton. Prof. Overton improves dairy health and production. *Cornell Daily Sun*, April 28. Available at http://cornellsun.com/node/42561. Accessed August 6, 2010.

Mathé, A. A. 1971. Decreased circulating epinephrine, possibly secondary to decreases hypothalamic-adrenal medullary discharge: A supplementary hypothesis of bronchial asthma pathogenesis. *Journal of Psychosomatic Research* 15(3):349-359.

Matsuoka, L. Y., J. Wortsman, J. G. Haddad, P. Kolm, and B. W. Hollis. 1991. Racial pigmentation and the cutaneous synthesis of vitamin D. *Archives of Dermatology* 127(4):536-538.

McCraty, R., B. Barrios-Choplin, D. Rozman, M. Atkinson, and A. D. Watkins. 1998. The impact of a new emotional self-management program on stress, emotions, heart rate variability, DHEA, and cortisol. *Integrative Psychological and Behavioral Science* 33(2):151-170.

McEwen, B. S. 2002. *The End of Stress as We Know It.* Washington, D.C.: Joseph Henry Press.

McEwen, B. S. 2005. Stressed or stressed out: What is the difference? *Journal of Psychiatry and Neuroscience* 30(5):315-318.

McEwen, B. S., C. A. Biron, K. W. Brunson, et al. 1996. The role of adrenocorticoids as modulators of immune function in health and disease: Neural, endocrine, and immune interactions. *Brain Research Reviews* 23(1-2):79-133.

Meikle, A. W., and F. H. Tyler. 1977. Potency and duration of action of glucocorticoids: Effects of hydrocortisone, prednisone, and dexamethasone on human pituitary-adrenal function. *American Journal of Medicine* 63(2):200-207.

Meissner, O., P. Mrozikiewicz, T. Bobkiewicz-Kozlowska, et al. 2006. Hormone-balancing effect of pre-gelatinized organic maca (*Lepidium peruvianum* Chacon): (I) Biochemical and pharmacodynamic study on maca using clinical laboratory model on ovariectomized rats. *International Journal of Biomedical Science* 2(3):260-272.

Mendelson, J., M. Ogata, and N. Mello. 1971. Adrenal function and alcoholism. *Psychosomatic Medicine* 33(2):145-157.

Merke, D. P., and G. B. Cutler. 1997. New approaches to the treatment of congenital adrenal hyperplasia. *Journal of the American Medical Association* 277(13):1073-1076.

Monteleone, P., M. Maj, L. Beinat, M. Natale, and D. Kemali. 1992. Blunting by chronic phosphatidylserine administration of the stress-induced activation of the hypothalamo-pituitary-adrenal axis in healthy men. *European Journal of Clinical Pharmacology* 42(4):385-388.

Mulatero, P., M. Stowasser, K. C. Loh, et al. 2004. Increased diagnosis of primary aldosteronism, including surgically correctable forms, in centers from five continents. *Journal of Clinical Endocrinology and Metabolism* 89(3):1045-1050.

Munck, A., P. M. Guyre, and N. J. Holbrook. 1984. Physiological functions of glucocorticoids in stress and their relation to pharmacological actions. *Endocrine Review* 5(1):25-44.

Nilzén, V., J. Babol, P. Dutta, N. Lundeheim, A. Enfält, and K. Lundström. 2001. Free range rearing of pigs with access to pasture grazing: Effect on fatty acid composition and lipid oxidation products. *Meat Science* 58(3):267-275.

Nocerino, E., M. Amato, and A. Izzo. 2000. The aphrodisiac and adaptogenic properties of ginseng. *Fitoterapia* 71(1):S1-S5.

Orentreich, N., J. Brind, R. Rizer, and J. Vogelman. 1984. Age changes and sex differences in serum dehydroepiandrosterone sulfate concentrations throughout adulthood. *Journal of Clinical Endocrinology and Metabolism* 59(3):551-555.

Panda, S., and A. Kar. 1998. Changes in thyroid hormone concentrations after administration of ashwagandha root extract to adult male mice. *Journal of Pharmacy and Pharmacology* 50(9):1065-1068.

Panda, S., and A. Kar. 1999. Gugulu (*Commiphora mukul*) induces triiodothyronine production: Possible involvement of lipid peroxidation. *Life Sciences* 65(12):137-141.

Peters, E., R. Anderson, D. Nieman, H. Fickl, and V. Jogessar. 2001. Vitamin C supplementation attenuates the increases in circulating cortisol, adrenaline, and anti-inflammatory polypeptides following ultra-marathon running. *International Journal of Sports Medicine* 22(7):537-543.

Puchacz, E., W. E. Stumpf, E. K. Stachowiak, and M. K. Stachowiak. 1996. Vitamin D increases expression of the tyrosine hydroxylase gene in adrenal medullary cells. *Molecular Brain Research* 36(1):193-196.

Putnam, J., J. Allshouse, and L. Kantor. 2002. U.S. per capita food supply trends: More calories, refined carbohydrates, and fats. *Food Review* (25)3:2-15.

Raber, J. 1998. Detrimental effects of chronic hypothalamic-pituitary-adrenal axis activation: From obesity to memory deficits. *Molecular Neurobiology* 18(1):1-22.

Raison, C., L. Capuron, and A. H. Miller. 2006. Cytokines sing the blues: Inflammation and the pathogenesis of depression. *Trends in Immunology* 27(1):24-31.

Rakoff-Nahoum, S. 2006. Why cancer and inflammation? *Yale Journal of Biology and Medicine* 79(3-4):123-130.

Reis, J., D. von Mühlen, E. Miller, E. Michos, and L. Appel. 2009. Vitamin D status and cardiometabolic risk factors in the United States adolescent population. *Pediatrics* 124(3):e371-379.

Rimmelea, U., B. Zellwegerb, B. Martic, et al. 2007. Trained men show lower cortisol, heart rate, and psychological responses to psychosocial stress compared with untrained men. *Psychoneuroendocrinology* 32(6):627-635.

Rosmond, R., M. F. Dallman, and P. Björntorp. 1998. Stress-related cortisol secretion in men: relationships with abdominal obesity and endocrine, metabolic, and hemodynamic abnormalities. *Journal of Clinical Endocrinology and Metabolism* 83(6):1853-1859.

Rothenberg, R., and K. Becker. 2007. *Forever Ageless.* Encinitas, CA: California HealthSpan Institute.

Sahin, Y., and F. Kelestimur. 1997. The frequency of late-onset 21-hydroxylase and 11-beta-hydroxylase deficiency in women with polycystic ovary syndrome. *European Journal of Endocrinology* 137(6):670-674.

Sapolsky, R. M. 1992. *Stress, the Aging Brain, and the Mechanisms of Neuron Death.* Cambridge, MA: MIT Press.

Scheier, M. F., and C. S. Carver. 1993. On the power of positive thinking: The benefits of being optimistic. *Current Directions in Psychological Science* 2(1):26-30.

Schleimer, R. 2000. Interactions between the hypothalamic-pituitary-adrenal axis and allergic inflammation. *Journal of Allergy and Clinical Immunology* 106(5 Suppl):S270-S274.

Schnall, S., K. Harber, J. Stefanucci, and D. Proffitt. 2008. Social support and the perception of geographical slant. *Journal of Experimental Social Psychology* 44(5):1246-1255.

Seltzer, L. J., T. E. Ziegler, and S. D. Pollak. 2010. Social vocalizations can release oxytocin in humans. *Proceedings of the Royal Society B: Biological Sciences* 77(1694):2661-2666.

Shealy, C. N. 1995. A review of dehydroepiandrosterone (DHEA). *Integrative Physiological and Behavioral Science* 30(4):308-313.

Sibbald, W. J., A. Short, M. P. Cohen, and R. F. Wilson. 1977. Variations in adrenocortical responsiveness during severe bacterial infections: Unrecognized adrenocortical insufficiency in severe bacterial infections. *Annals of Surgery* 186(1):29-33.

Simopoulos, P. 2002. Omega-3 fatty acids in inflammation and autoimmune diseases. *Journal of the American College of Nutrition* 21(6):495-505.

Simopoulos, A., and N. Salem. 1992. Egg yolk as a source of long-chain polyunsaturated fatty acids in infant feeding. *American Journal of Clinical Nutrition* 55(2):411-414.

Singh, N., R. Nath, A. Lata, S. P. Singh, R. P. Kohli, and K. P. Bhargava. 1982. *Withania somnifera* (ashwagandha), a rejuvenating herbal drug which enhances survival during stress (an adaptogen). *International Journal of Crude Drug Research* 20(1):29-35.

Smith, P., D. Martino, Z. Cai, et al. 2007. Agriculture. In *Climate Change 2007: Mitigation. Contribution of Working Group III to the Fourth Assessment Report of the Intergovernmental Panel on Climate Change*, edited by B. Metz, O. R. Davidson, P. R. Bosch, et al. Cambridge, UK: Cambridge University Press.

Standing Committee on the Scientific Evaluation of Dietary Reference Intakes, Food and Nutrition Board, Institute of Medicine. 1997. *Dietary Reference Intakes for Calcium, Phosphorus, Magnesium, Vitamin D, and Fluoride.* Washington, D.C.: National Academy Press.

Stansbury, K., and M. R. Gunnar. 1994. Adrenocortical activity and emotion regulation. *Monographs of the Society for Research in Child Development* 59(2-3):108-134.

Steptoe, A., E. L. Gibson, R. Vuononvirta, et al. 2007. The effects of tea on psychophysiological stress responsivity and post-stress recovery: A randomised double-blind trial. *Psychopharmacology* 190(1):81-89.

Stokes, P. E. 1995. The potential role of excessive cortisol induced by HPA hyperfunction in the pathogenesis of depression. *European Neuropsychopharmacology* 5(1):77-82.

Straub, R. H., J. Schölmerich, and B. Zietz. 2000. Replacement therapy with DHEA plus corticosteroids in patients with chronic inflammatory diseases: Substitutes of adrenal and sex hormones. *Zeitschrift für Rheumatologie* 59(Suppl 2):II108-II118.

Straub, R. H., D. Vogl, V. Gross, B. Lang, J. Schölmerich, and T. Andus. 1998. Association of humoral markers of inflammation and dehydroepiandrosterone sulfate or cortisol serum levels in patients with chronic inflammatory bowel disease. *American Journal of Gastroenterology* 93(11):2197-2202.

Tanizawa, H., H. Numano, T. Odani, Y. Takino, T. Hayashi, and S. Arichi. 1981. Study of the saponin of *Panax ginseng* C. A. Meyer. I. Inhibitory effect on adrenal atrophy, thymus atrophy, and the decrease of serum potassium ion concentration induced by cortisone acetate in unilaterally adrenalectomized rats. *Journal of the Pharmaceutical Society of Japan* 101:169-173.

Tarasov, I., V. Sheibak, and A. Moiseenok. 1985. Adrenal cortex functional activity in pantothenate deficiency and the administration of the vitamin or its derivatives. *Voprosy Pitaniia* 4:51-54.

Traustadottir, T., P. R. Bosch, and K. S. Matt. 2005. The HPA axis response to stress in women: Effects of aging and fitness. *Psychoneuroendocrinology* 30(4):392-402.

U.S. Department of Agriculture. 2002. *Agriculture Fact Book 2001–2002.* Washington, DC: Government Printing Office.

Vasto, S., G. Candore, F. Listì, et al. 2008. Inflammation, genes, and zinc in Alzheimer's disease. *Brain Research Reviews* 58(1):96-105.

Vgontzas, A. N., C. Tsigos, E. O. Bixler, et al. 1998. Chronic insomnia and activity of the stress system: A preliminary study. *Journal of Psychosomatic Research* 45(1):21-31.

Vicennati, V., L. Ceroni, L. Gagliardi, A. Gambineri, and R. Pasquali. 2002. Response of the hypothalamic-pituitary-adrenocortical axis to high-protein/fat and high-carbohydrate meals in women with different obesity phenotypes. *Journal of Clinical Endocrinology and Metabolism* 87(8):3984-3988,

Virchow, R. 1860. *Cellular Pathology as Based upon Physiological and Pathological Histology*. London: Churchill.

Weill, S., D. Chesneau, and L. Safraou. 2002. Effects of introducing linseed in livestock diet on blood fatty acid composition of consumers of animal products. *Annals of Nutrition and Metabolism* 46(5):182-191.

Whitworth, J., P. Williamson, G. Mangos, and J. Kelly. 2005. Cardiovascular consequences of cortisol excess. *Journal of Vascular Health and Risk Management* 1(4):291-299.

Wilson, D., D. Foster, H. Kronenberg, and P. Larsen. 1998. *Williams Textbook of Endocrinology*. Philadelphia: W. B. Saunders.

Wilson, J. 2001. *Adrenal Fatigue: The 21st-Century Stress Syndrome*. Petaluma, CA: Smart Publications.

Yang, Q., Y. Hang, and D. Sun. 2001. Effect of combined drug-acupuncture anesthesia on hypothalamo-pituitary-adrenocortical axis response and glucose metabolism in open-heart surgery patients. *Chinese Journal of Integrated Traditional and Western Medicine* 21(10):729-731.

Yehuda, R., M. Teicher, J. Seckl, R. Grossman, A. Morris, and L. Bierer. 2007. Parental posttraumatic stress disorder as a vulnerability factor for low cortisol trait in offspring of Holocaust survivors. *Archives of General Psychiatry* 64(9):1040-1048.

Yetley, E. A. 2008. Assessing the vitamin D status of the U.S. population. *American Journal of Clinical Nutrition* 88(2):558S-564S.

Zisapel, N., R. Tarrasch, and M. Laudon. 2005. The relationship between melatonin and cortisol rhythms Clinical implications of melatonin therapy. *Drug Development Research* 65(3):119-125.

About the Author

Kathryn R. Simpson, MS, was an executive in the biotech industry when she was diagnosed with multiple sclerosis. Research led her to discover that her symptoms were caused by multiple hormonal deficiencies—including low adrenal and thyroid hormone levels. She resolved all of her debilitating symptoms by rebuilding her adrenal function and supplementing low hormone levels.

Simpson received a bachelor's degree from Ohio Wesleyan University and a masters of science degree from the University of Southern California. She founded a specialty hormone clinic to treat hormone imbalance and diseases such as multiple sclerosis, lupus, and fibromyalgia. Today, it is dedicated to ongoing endocrine research and education. Simpson is CEO of Cerulean Pharmaceutical, which researches and develops therapies for the treatment of endocrine-related disorders. She is author of *The Perimenopause and Menopause Workbook*, *The MS Solution*, and *The Women's Guide to Thyroid Health*, and lives in Los Olivos, CA, with her husband, Robert, and three sons, Tyler, Kyle, and Myles.

Other Books by Kathryn R. Simpson

The Perimenopause and Menopause Workbook: A Comprehensive, Personalized Guide to Hormone Health for Women (with Dale E. Bredesen). Oakland, CA: New Harbinger Publications, 2006.

The MS Solution: How I Solved the Puzzle of My Multiple Sclerosis. Santa Ynez, CA: Los Olivos Publishing, 2008.

The Women's Guide to Thyroid Health: Comprehensive Solutions for All Your Thyroid Symptoms. Oakland, CA: New Harbinger Publications, 2009.

Index

cortisol: bioidentical, 50, 75–76; brain function and, 30; causes of excessive, 22–23; chronic health problems and, 17–18; effects of deficient, 45–47; effects of excessive, 28–32; immune system and, 16, 29; inflammation and, 2, 16; physiological functions of, 8–9, 10; production patterns of, 10–12; reducing excess production of, 68–72; relationship between adrenaline and, 9; sleep problems and, 22, 31; stress response and, 5, 6; synthetic forms of, 38; testing levels of, 55–57; thyroid function and, 83; weight gain and, 10, 29

CRH (corticotropin-releasing hormone), 15; CRH stimulation test, 59–60

Cushing's disease, 23

D

deep breathing, 118–119

depression, 31

DHEA (dehydroepiandrosterone), 12, 13, 77; effects of deficient, 47–48; effects of excessive, 32; supplemental, 77; testing levels of, 58

DHT (dihydrotestosterone), 62

diabetes, 8, 29, 57

diet, 95–107; anti-inflammatory, 95; case example of changing, 102–103; cortisol production and, 22; food allergies/sensitivities and, 105; general guidelines for, 97–107; key points about, 108; water consumption and, 104. *See also* eating habits; foods

digestive enzymes, 73

doctors: choosing experienced, 53; resources for locating, 125–126

dopamine, 47

drugs. *See* medications

E

eating habits, 95–108; dietary guidelines, 97–107; pattern of meals and snacks, 96; quantity of food consumed, 96–97; slow, mindful eating, 107. *See also* diet; foods

emotional imbalances, 31

emotional support, 115

endocrine system: adrenal glands and, 13–15; stress hormone production and, 23, 30; testing for imbalances in, 61–64

energy level, 45

environmental toxins, 23

essential fatty acids (EFAs), 100

estradiol, 61, 62

estrogen, 23, 61, 62

exercise: adrenal fatigue and, 113; caution about overdoing, 112; cortisol production and, 22; stress management and, 111–113

exhaustion, 11, 45

F

fatigue. *See* adrenal fatigue

fats, 99–102; omega-3 and omega-6, 100; saturated, 100–101; trans or hydrogenated, 101–102

female sex hormones, 61–62

fiber, 97, 98–99

fibrinogen, 29

fibromyalgia, 50

fight-or-flight reaction, 5, 109, 110

financial worries, 114

fish oil, 69

fludrocortisone, 78

follicle-stimulating hormone (FSH), 62

foods: allergies/sensitivities to, 105; carbohydrates, 97–99; fats, 99–102; importance of chewing, 107; processed, 104–105; proteins, 102; soy products, 105. *See also* diet; eating habits

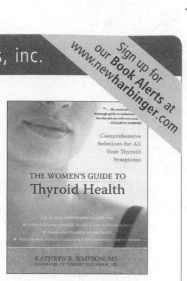
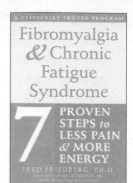
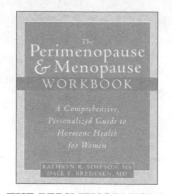
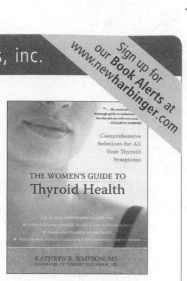
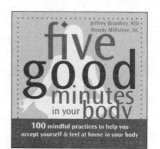
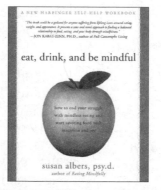
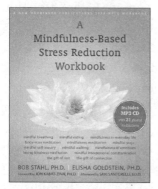